The Flexible
Stretching Strap

WORKBOOK

The Flexible
Stretching Strap
WORKBOOK

Step-by-Step Techniques
for Maximizing Your Range of Motion and Flexibility

Mark Kovacs, PhD, FACSM, CSCS*D, MTPS

ULYSSES PRES

Published in the United States by
Ulysses Press
P.O. Box 3440
Berkeley, CA 94703
www.ulyssespress.com

ISBN: 978-1-61243-367-7
Library of Congress Control Number 2014932310

Printed in the United Stares by Bang Printing
10 9 8 7 6 5 4 3 2 1

Acquisitions: Kelly Reed
Managing editor: Claire Chun
Editors: Lauren Harrison, Lily Chou
Proofreader: Renee Rutledge
Indexer: Sayre Van Young
Front cover and interior design: what!design @ whatweb.com
Cover artwork: woman © Rapt Productions; horizontal strap graphic © sellingpix/shutterstock.com
Interior photographs: © Rapt Productions except on page 12 © Photobank gallery/shutterstock.com
Models: Kathleen Aeschlimann, Mark Kovacs, Toni Silver
Make-up: Sabrina Foster

Distributed by Publishers Group West

PLEASE NOTE: This book has been written and published strictly for informational purposes, and in no way should be used as a substitute for consultation with health care professionals. You should not consider educational material herein to be the practice of medicine or to replace consultation with a physician or other medical practitioner. The author and publisher are providing you with information in this work so that you can have the knowledge and can choose, at your own risk, to act on that knowledge. The author and publisher also urge all readers to be aware of their health status and to consult health care professionals before beginning any health program.

This book is independently authored and published. No sponsorship or endorsement of this book by, and no affiliation with any flexible stretching strap, including the TheraBand™ Stretch Strap or any other trademarked brands or products mentioned or pictured, is claimed or suggested. All trademarks that appear in this book belong to their respective owners and are used here for informational purposes only. The author and publisher encourage readers to patronize the quality brands and other products mentioned and pictured in this book.

TABLE OF CONTENTS

PART 1

Getting Started

INTRODUCTION

A typical day for a college athlete involves hours of practice, then weight workouts often followed by rehabilitation or injury prevention work and recovery (i.e., massage treatment by a physical therapist, athletic trainer or chiropractor). A mom, on the other hand, bends down constantly to pick up her child. Even recreational adult tennis players put strain on their bodies during practice and matches. Our bodies are constantly being pulled, pushed, stressed and generally worn out. Sports and activities of daily living cause muscles to contract on a regular basis. These contractions can shorten certain muscles and over time can reduce those muscles' range of motion. Fortunately, many factors help our bodies recover, adapt and improve. Stretching is one of the best methods to ease stress, reduce negative effects of heavy training and improve overall performance.

Adding regular stretching to the weekly routine can significantly improve flexibility and serve to provide many health, wellness and performance benefits to athletes at all levels, from recreational to professional. It's also essential for any athlete who's rehabbing from surgery or an extended layoff due to injury.

As a performance physiologist, strength and conditioning coach and personal trainer, I've worked with thousands of athletes, ranging from recreational sports enthusiasts to some of the best athletes in the world, such as Olympians and NFL, NBA and MLB players. I've implemented effective flexibility programs into the daily routine of these athletes. One of the most important aspects in building these workouts is to keep in mind that not all athletes need the same stretching program. Some require a lower-body focus, while some need more upper-body work; certain sports need extra focus on rotational movements in the core/trunk area, whereas other sports need significant time spent on reducing major flexibility imbalances.

Each athlete is different, as is each sport. Fortunately, some common flexibility exercises overlap for certain sports. For example, a baseball pitcher and tennis player both have reduced range of motion in their dominant shoulder—specifically, the internal range of motion. This is a common result of the demands of their sports. As a result, baseball and tennis players should perform a specific stretching routine to help limit the likelihood of this decreased range of motion. This is just one example of a sport-specific flexibility limitation that occurs due to the thousands of hours of training and competition that athletes—at all levels—endure.

Using the flexible stretching strap can significantly increase range of motion above and beyond general stretching alone. This book will provide an effective, portable and efficient method to stretch all the major muscles of the body using this simple yet highly useful tool.

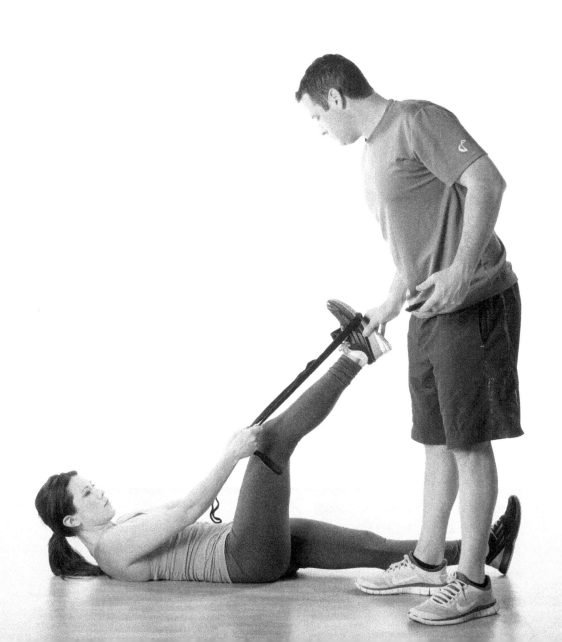

GETTING TO KNOW YOUR BODY

Flexibility is at the base of all good human movement. If you have limited flexibility (range of motion) in a particular area of the body, plane of motion or single muscle or joint, you'll be limited in achieving optimal movement in sports or daily life. This limitation can restrict performance and increase overall imbalances, and over time can potentially lead to injury. It's important to appropriately work on flexibility in a progressive manner and in a way that will improve your performance in sports and in activities of daily living.

The human body is a unique structure. It's made up of more than 640 muscles and approximately 206 major bones, and is packed within a tissue known as fascia that's connected from head to toe. Having appropriate flexibility and understanding how to effectively improve flexibility can make a major difference in your life and lead to better performance in your sport (or sports) of choice.

Body Movements

This book is designed to help you on your journey to improved flexibility. To get the most out of it, you should be familiar with some basic stretching vocabulary. The following are some of the most frequently used terms with respect to flexibility, and will provide a good overview to help you navigate the terminology throughout the remainder of the book.

Range of Motion

Range of motion is the degree of movement that occurs at a joint. For athletes, it's important to have functional or sport-specific range of motion in the planes of motion and movement patterns used during practice or competition. A hockey goalie, for example, needs a much greater range of motion in the hip than a 100-meter track sprinter. These differences are determined by the demands of the sport. The hockey goalie needs to drop and spread his legs dozens of times per training or competition day, and he needs to train to successfully accomplish this movement. The sprinter, on the other hand, only needs to successfully run in a straight line (albeit very quickly). The demands of the activities are very different and how those athletes train, recover and stretch will be different as a result.

For individuals who are focused on improving activities of daily living, the appropriate range of motion allows for optimum function during normal life. For example, those who have to get into and out of a car or truck multiple times per day need the flexibility in the core/trunk area, as well as the lower body, to effectively accomplish this. Without performing regularly structured stretching exercises, this seemingly simple task of getting into and out of a vehicle can become challenging over time and can result in tightness, pain and injury over an extended period.

Flexibility

Flexibility is the measure of range of motion and has both static and dynamic components. **Static flexibility** is the range of movement around a joint and its surrounding muscles, ligaments and connective tissue during a passive movement. Static flexibility requires no voluntary muscle activity, meaning the stretch is produced from an external source, such as a partner, gravity or a machine. For example, one of the most traditional static stretching exercises is when you sit on the ground with your legs extended and try to reach forward to touch your toes and hold the stretch for 30 seconds.

Dynamic flexibility is the available range of motion during active movements and therefore requires voluntary muscle actions. An athlete's range of motion is typically greater dynamically than statically because the athlete uses movement to help initiate the exercise. Think about a walking lunge. This is sometimes considered a strength-training exercise, but it's also a dynamic flexibility movement. If no added resistance is provided (in addition to bodyweight), then the exercise involves the individual stretching of the hips and lower body during each step that's taken.

The Muscles of Your Body

To greatly improve your understanding of how best to stretch to improve performance, it's important to have a basic understanding of the different muscles of the body. The following section summarizes the major muscles, as well as their location, basic function and some movements that use these muscles the most. It must be understood that in most movements in sports and daily living, multiple muscle groups are used simultaneously; in sports especially, it's rare that a single muscle alone will be responsible for most movements.

The **trapezius** is a large muscle in the upper back and neck area that helps move your head and connect it to the shoulders. When you feel "knots" in your neck and shoulders, that discomfort is usually in your trapezius. Exercises like upright rows and shoulder shrugs recruit the traps.

All shoulder movement, especially anything involving overhead lifting, uses the **deltoids**, the largest muscle group of the shoulder. The deltoids are composed of three parts: anterior, posterior and medial. Any time you "use your arms," your deltoids are working. Push-ups, bench presses, and side and rear arm raises all work the deltoids.

Any time you move your hand toward your shoulder, you're using your **biceps**, the muscles located on the front of the upper arm. Lifting movements, especially with palms up, like biceps curls, use the biceps, as do upper-body and back exercises involving pulling movements.

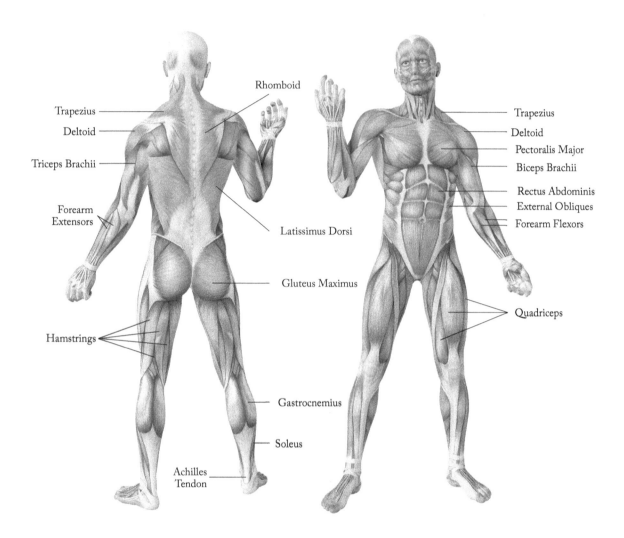

The **pectoralis** muscles are on the front of the upper chest. They pull the shoulder and arm forward, meaning you use them to push up from a lying position, as in a push-up, or to push open something like a door, somewhat like performing a bench press.

The **latissimus dorsi** and **rhomboids** are the major muscles of the back. The rhomboids are located between the shoulder blades, while the lats are the large triangular muscle in the midback. Developed lats give your body that classic V shape, making your waist appear smaller. Together these muscles help with postural alignment (i.e., keeping your shoulders back) and upper-body pulling movements, like opening a door. Chin-ups, pull-ups and lateral pull-downs will work your lats, and exercises like chin-ups and bent-arm rows are more focused on the rhomboids.

The **erector spinae** is sometimes called the "lower back" muscle, although it runs up your entire back. Like the lats, this muscle helps with postural alignment. You can strengthen it through back extensions.

The **obliques**, part of the core/trunk muscles located on the sides of the body, help with rotation and side flexion (bending) of the body. For strong internal and external oblique muscles to ward off back pain, perform twisting crunches as part of your regular exercise program.

Made up of several muscles (gluteus maximus, medius and minimus, as well as the tensor fascia latae) the **gluteus** is used for most everyday activities like walking, standing up, and climbing stairs. The gluteus maximus is one of the strongest muscles in the body and can be developed and strengthened with classic exercises like squats, lunges and leg presses.

The **hamstrings** are made up of three muscles: the semitendinosus, semimembranosus and biceps femoris. Simply put, they're the muscles on the back of the thigh. Used for movements as basic as walking, the hamstrings can be improved through deep lunges, deadlifts, and leg curls.

Working in opposition to the hamstrings are the **quadriceps**, located on the front of the thigh. The quads are made up of four muscles, including the rectus femoris, vastus lateralis, vastus medialis and vastus intermedius. Squats, lunges and leg presses will all help strengthen the quads, which are recruited every time you stand up, walk and climb stairs.

Collectively known as the **calves**, the gastro-cnemius and soleus are located on the back of the lower legs. The gastrocnemius gives your lower leg a rounded shape; the soleus is underneath the gastrocnemius. Both standing and seated calf raises work this muscle pair, which you use every day to push off for walking or standing on your tiptoes.

WHAT IS STRETCHING?

Stretching means many different things to different people. In the simplest terms, stretching is defined as "to make something wider or longer without tearing or breaking it." This is accurate when discussing general stretching for sports or activities for daily living. However, the science of stretching has exploded over the past decade, and many different techniques have been researched and dozens more have been tried in gyms, athletic training facilities, and strength and conditioning environments worldwide. A number of different techniques have been shown to improve range of motion, and this book will focus on a few that have been shown to specifically improve flexibility in athletes and regular individuals alike.

Many misconceptions exist about the best ways to stretch, but two aspects need to occur to have an effective stretching program: 1) a gradual increase in functional range of motion; and 2) a safe (low injury risk) method to achieve this increased range of motion. Increasing range of motion alone is not very challenging; however, increasing it in a safe, efficient and practical manner should be the goal. This book uses the flexible stretching strap to help achieve these goals.

Much research has been performed looking at the best ways and times to stretch for improved athletic performance and also to increase general range of motion. Dynamic stretching exercises have been shown to be highly beneficial before physical activity, whereas static flexibility exercises are preferred post-exercise as they can improve range of motion in a safe manner. However, if exercise is performed immediately following static stretching, individuals see a short-term reduction in strength, speed and power. The mechanisms behind this phenomena are still being investigated, but the reasons link back to a concept that a stretched muscle which is not also producing force during the stretching (which is the case during dynamic stretching) will have less ability to transfer force, resulting in less strength, speed and power. Therefore, static stretching is not recommended immediately before exercise.

The exercises provided throughout this book use a flexible stretching strap, which can aid in traditional static stretching exercises, but the use of the strap can also allow for all the exercises to be performed more dynamically (stretching while moving). These terms—dynamic and static—will be described in more detail in the next section.

Types of Stretching

There are three different (broad) types of stretching: static, dynamic and ballistic.

STATIC STRETCHING: This is a constant stretch held at an end point for anywhere between 10 seconds and 5 minutes. This is what most people traditionally think of when the term "stretching" is used. However, as can be seen below, stretching can involve a lot more.

DYNAMIC STRETCHING: This functional stretching utilizes sport-specific (or activity-specific) movements to prepare the body for activity. Dynamic stretching focuses on movement patterns requiring a combination of muscles, joints and planes of motion, whereas static stretching typically focuses on a single muscle group, joint and plane of motion.

BALLISTIC STRETCHING: This involves active muscle effort and uses a bouncing-type movement to increase the range without holding the stretch at an end position. Unlike static stretching, ballistic stretching triggers the stretch reflex (page 17). You see this frequently in less-experienced athletes, who, for example, may try to touch their toes by bouncing up and down to reach lower, putting a lot of strain on the lower back. Ballistic stretching is typically not recommended as a component of an effective warm-up for the vast majority of the population. It should be avoided by individuals with a history of lower back and/or hamstring injuries.

Other Terms

CONCENTRIC CONTRACTION: A contraction that involves the shortening of the muscle, such as the upward phase of a biceps curl.

ECCENTRIC CONTRACTION: When tension is increased on a muscle as it's lengthened (sometimes also called eccentric muscle action), such as the downward phase of a biceps curl.

ISOMETRIC CONTRACTION: When a muscle contracts without changing length, such as the static hold of the biceps curl anywhere during the movement.

KINETIC CHAIN: A combination of several successively arranged joints constituting the total system. From a human anatomy perspective, think of this as all the major joints in the body starting at the ankle and going all the way up through the chain to the neck and arms.

OPEN-CHAIN MOVEMENT: When the end of the anatomical segment can move freely. Think of a leg extension exercise where the foot can move freely.

CLOSED-CHAIN MOVEMENT: When the end of the segment cannot move freely; typically this is the result of it being in contact with an immovable object. For example, a squat or lunge is a closed-chain movement in that the end of the segment (foot/ankle) is in contact with the ground (immovable object).

ROTATIONAL STRENGTH: When an appropriate amount of strength can be maintained during a rotational movement. A good example is swinging a golf club, when the lower body is stable and the upper body rotates around the axis of the body.

SUPINE: Lying face-up on your back.

PRONE: Lying face-down on your stomach.

FLEXION: A bending movement around a joint that decreases the angle between the bones of the limb at the joint, such as when bending the elbow.

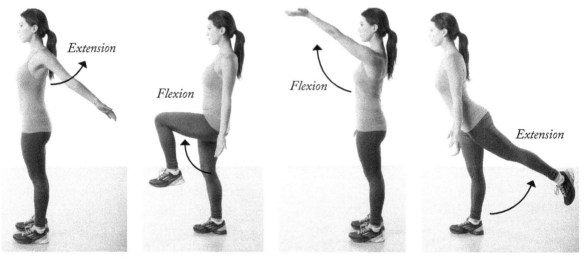

Angular movements: flexion and extension at the shoulder and hip

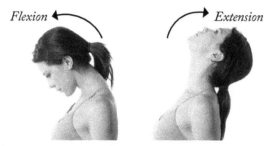

Angular movements: flexion and extension of the neck

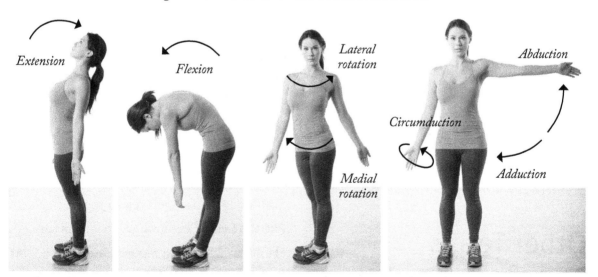

Angular movements: flexion and
extension of the vertical column

Rotation of the torso

Angular movements: abduction,
adduction and circumduction of the
upper limb at the shoulder

THE FLEXIBLE STRETCHING STRAP WORKBOOK

EXTENSION: The opposite of flexion—a straightening movement that increases the angle between body parts, such as when you stand up (your knees extend).

INTERNAL ROTATION: Rotation toward the center of the body. This can be accomplished at many joints, most commonly the shoulder and hip.

EXTERNAL ROTATION: Rotation away from the center of the body. This can be accomplished at many joints, most commonly the shoulder and hip.

PLANTAR FLEXION: Movement of the foot downward (pointing your toes).

DORSIFLEXION: Movement of the foot upward (flexing your foot).

The Stretch Reflex

The stretch reflex is an important term to understand. Sometimes called the myotatic or knee-jerk reflex, the stretch reflex is an automated response by the body to a stretch stimulus in the muscle. When a muscle spindle is stretched, an impulse is sent to the spinal cord and then a response is sent back to the muscle telling it to contract. Since the impulse only has to go to the spinal cord and back, not all the way to the brain, it's a very quick impulse, generally occurring in 1–2 milliseconds. Think of this as a safety mechanism in the body. It's designed as a protective measure to prevent muscles from tearing. When the muscle is stretched to a large degree, the impulse sent back to the muscle is to immediately contract the muscle to protect it from being pulled forcefully or beyond a normal (safe) range.

At the same time, the stretch reflex has an inhibitory aspect to the opposing (antagonist) muscles. When the stretch reflex is activated, a signal to contract is sent to the stretched muscle, while a signal to relax is sent to the opposing muscles. For example, when stretching the hamstring muscles, the quadriceps muscles relax. Without this inhibitory action, as soon as the stretched muscle begins to contract, the opposing muscle would be stretched, causing a stretch reflex in that one. Both muscles would end up contracting simultaneously.

Another example of the stretch reflex is the knee-jerk test performed by physicians. When the patellar tendon is tapped with a small hammer or other device, it causes a slight stretch in the tendon, and consequently the quadriceps muscles. The result is a quick, although mild, contraction of the quadriceps muscles, resulting in a small kicking motion.

The stretch reflex is also very important in helping maintain proper posture. A slight lean to either side causes a stretch in the spinal, hip and leg muscles, and those same muscles on the other side are signaled to relax to regain balance. This is a constant process of adjusting and maintaining that happens subconsciously. The body is constantly under push and pull forces from slight muscle imbalances in strength and flexibility, as well as from gravity. Having an effective stretching program can make positive adaptations to allow for improvements.

BENEFITS OF STRETCHING WITH THE FLEXIBLE STRETCHING STRAP

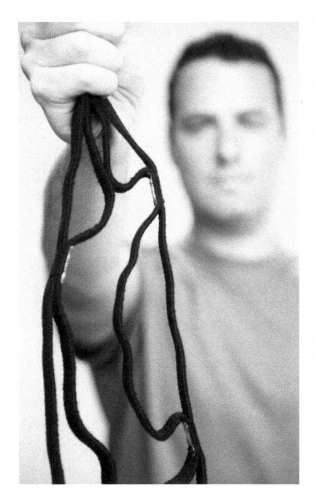

There are many benefits of strap-free stretching. However, if you add the flexible stretching strap to your traditional stretches, it won't be long before you see increased flexibility and range of motion. While supporting classic static stretches, the strap also allows for dynamic stretches, including multiple contract/relax-type stretching routines. These variations involve contracting and relaxing the muscle that's being stretched to help increase range of motion at a faster rate.

The strap's multiple loops also permit gradual stretching of major muscle groups with safety, control and efficacy. It eliminates the need for a partner or gym access to an expensive stretching machine.

Think about traditional static stretching, such as touching your toes and holding for 30 seconds. It's beneficial—it can increase range of motion, is rather easy to perform, can be performed nearly anywhere and is a relatively safe activity. Most people feel like stretching is a good activity and can help in many respects, yet most people (especially active ones) don't perform as much flexibility training as they'd like to (or should!).

It's similar to overall exercise programs and good nutrition plans: Most people know they'd like to do a better job in these areas, but for many reasons do not achieve the results as effectively as they'd like to. You might put off a traditional static stretching program because it's rather time-consuming (e.g., hold each stretch for 30 seconds to 3 minutes and repeat multiple times per muscle group) and the sensation of holding a stretch for an extended period of time is often uncomfortable (many people may say painful). To see noticeable improvements in range of motion takes many weeks, if not months. All these factors contribute to numerous people not performing regular flexibility routines, or feeling like the routines they're performing may not be achieving their desired flexibility goals.

However, using the flexible stretching strap can help mitigate many of these common complaints:

1) It allows you to reach a greater range of motion in traditional static stretching movements. It also allows the rest of your body to be more relaxed than if you weren't using the strap. See the photos below to note the difference between a stretch performed with and without the flexible stretching strap.

2) It can result in less discomfort while stretching if using a technique that involves only holding the stretched muscle for approximately 2 seconds. See page 20 for more information on this stretching technique, known as active isolated stretching (AIS).

3) It can be used as a long lever, requiring less effort to achieve a greater range of motion, compared to traditional static stretching.

4) It's portable, cost-effective and can help improve flexibility anywhere. It also has a variety of loops, which is very beneficial when stretching in different directions and also allows for different body parts to be secure while going through the various ranges of motion.

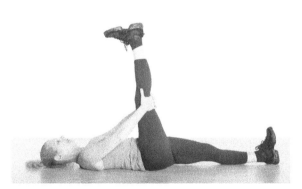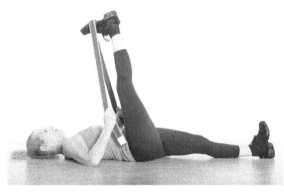

Lying hamstring stretch without and with the flexible stretching strap.

HOW TO STRETCH

Although many techniques exist to improve range of motion, this book will showcase some of the most well-defined and well-researched methods to help improve flexibility. Most exercises described throughout this book have three distinct phases that will serve as the baseline method for instruction for the different exercises. Use this basic three-part stretching sequence as a starting point. Depending on your specific needs, you can then progress to variations on the basic method, which are discussed later in this section.

1. Start Phase

• Begin by positioning your entire body in the appropriate position to allow for low to moderate tension in the strap.

2. Contract Phase

• Provide enough slack in the strap to support resistance during the muscle contraction.

• The muscle should be mid-range or slightly lengthened (elongated) depending on the type of stretch being performed.

• Contract the muscle through the range of motion or hold a static contraction for a few seconds (2–6 seconds). This phase allows for the initial muscle to be contracted and helps

achieve a greater stretch during the stretch phase than just stretching and holding for an arbitrary length of time.

3. Stretch Phase

• Provide enough tension in the strap to elongate (lengthen) the muscle.

• Hold the stretch for the appropriate time (2–30 seconds depending on the type of stretch).

Repeat this sequence 3–10 times (depending on the type and objectives of the stretch).

In addition to this basic stretching technique, there are other methods that can be used to add variation, which may be appropriate for different stretching goals.

Active Isolated Stretching (AIS)

When using active isolated stretching (AIS), you don't hold a stretch for 30 seconds to 3 minutes as you would in traditional static stretching. Instead, using the flexible stretching strap to assist you allows you to stretch your muscle slightly farther than your body would normally allow. This form of stretching results in greater gains as the muscle(s) go through a larger range of motion, so you see faster improvements in flexibility.

The stretches are held for only approximately 2 seconds and are performed for multiple repetitions. This avoids triggering the stretch reflex, which can be a limiting factor in improvement in athletic environments, injury rehabilitation or the desire to improve flexibility and function in the body. (For more on the stretch reflex, see page 17.)

Stretches performed with the AIS technique are "active," meaning you actually help move your own body part with your own muscles before any assistance with a strap (if done alone) or a coach/therapist (if assisted by coach/therapist) is initiated.

This active movement causes reciprocal inhibition, which occurs during a process when muscle(s) on one side of a joint relax to accommodate contraction on the other side of that joint. Joints are controlled by two opposing sets of muscles, extensors (which lengthen) and flexors (which contract), that must work together for smooth and efficient movement. When a muscle spindle is stretched and the stretch reflex is activated, the opposing muscle group must be inhibited to prevent it from working against the resulting contraction of the preferred muscle. This inhibition is accomplished by the actions of an interneuron in the spinal cord.

To think about this in a practical sense, take the common example of touching your toes. When you touch your toes to stretch your hamstring you're attempting to increase the stretch in the hamstrings group (lengthening the hamstrings muscles). For this to be accomplished successfully, the opposing (antagonist) muscles

start to relax. These opposing muscles are the quadriceps and, if they didn't start to relax, they'd limit the increased range that could be achieved while stretching the hamstring. This can be improved with different contract-relax techniques described on page 22.

Three Major Benefits of AIS

1) Limits the myotatic stretch reflex by holding the stretch for no more than approximately 2 seconds.

2) Encourages contraction of opposing muscles to allow the target muscle to relax. For example, when stretching the hamstrings, the quadriceps muscles on the front of the leg are contracted, relaxing the hamstrings and making them more susceptible to stretching. You'd lie on your back, lift your leg by using the muscles on the front of the leg, stretch the hamstrings by lightly pulling the leg back via the flexible stretching strap to the point of tightness for 2 seconds, then releasing.

3) The "assisted" aspect, in which the muscle is "helped" through the last few degrees of functional motion either by the coach/trainer/therapist or, more commonly, the flexible stretching strap.

Proprioceptive Neuromuscular Facilitation (PNF)

An active proprioceptive neuromuscular facilitation stretch involves a shortening contraction of the opposing muscle to stretch the target muscle. This is followed by an isometric contraction (a contraction that doesn't change the muscle's length) of the target muscle for a few seconds and is then followed by a relaxation of the muscle, which allows for a greater increase in range of motion.

There are three methods of PNF stretching:

CONTRACT-RELAX: This basic PNF stretch allows muscles to go through a greater range of motion than they might with the basic start-contract-stretch method. To contract-relax, stretch the muscle for at least 3 seconds at only 20–50% maximum effort to avoid muscle fatigue and injury. Then relax the muscle and activate its opposing muscle to stretch even further. The muscle you're stretching can then relax even more, allowing for that greater range of motion.

HOLD-RELAX: Very similar to the contract-relax technique, this is utilized when the muscle that's trying to be stretched is weak and cannot be activated properly. A progressive technique, this allows you to increase range of motion without the effort of the contract-relax technique. Your restricted muscle is put in a position of stretch followed by an isometric contraction. After holding the stretch for a time (3–30 seconds, depending on the purpose of the stretch), the restricted muscle is moved to a position of greater stretch.

CONTRACT-RELAX-ANTAGONIST/(AGONIST)-CONTRACT: This technique is performed by a stretch of the muscle (agonist), followed by a significant isometric contraction (near 100% of maximum) of the muscle and then stretching it even further. After that, maximum isometric contraction of the opposing muscle (antagonist) is performed, followed by another increase in the range of motion. For example, when stretching the hamstrings (agonist), the quadriceps muscles will be the antagonist.

Playing It Safe

One of the best uses of this book is to help learn and continually refine the technique of each exercise. This guide provides photos and written

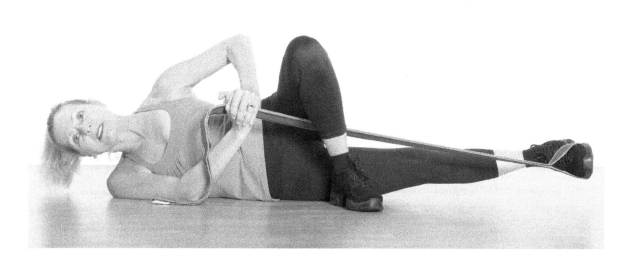

instructions on how to perform each stretch and movement pattern. It's easy for many athletes, especially young athletes, to go through the motions and not focus on correct technique. Without a focus on technique, you may not achieve the many benefits of a structured flexibility program. It's important to focus on "feeling" the muscles that are the focus of each stretch and consciously attempt to recruit those muscles. Technique is very important in these movements as it will help develop the correct muscles and movement patterns, but it will also limit the likelihood of injury. So take up the challenge and make your flexibility routines an integral part of your exercise or sport session. Remember to make sure that you have clearance from a medical professional before starting any type of exercise program, including a stretching program as outlined in this book.

Note that the stretches outlined here can be performed before or after exercise, or at other times throughout the day. It's preferable to perform the majority of the flexible stretching strap sequences at the end of the physical activity or during other specific stretching sections. However, if these stretches are performed before physical activity or sports performance, it's highly recommended that they're performed in a dynamic fashion. This means that the contract phases are held for less than 2 seconds, allowing for more movement in the stretch.

PART 2

The Programs

HOW TO USE THIS BOOK

This part of the book provides more than two dozen sample sport- and life-specific flexibility programs to help you focus on exercises to use for specific activities. The methods of stretching outlined in the previous section provide many variations to help you achieve your flexibility goals and objectives. In Part 3, you'll find dozens of exercises for the entire body, with photos and written descriptions using the start-contract-stretch format as the starting guide. However, for each of these stretches you can also advance to any of the three different variations of the PNF stretches outlined on page 21. As mentioned, the PNF stretches are progressive and require a little more effort and technique to perform effectively; they should be used as a progression once the three-step process is mastered and a comfort level exists with using this technique.

For all programs, the number of repetitions varies by experience level. Beginners should do 5 reps of each stretch. Intermediate stretchers should perform 10 reps, and more advanced athletes can do 15 reps of each stretch.

ACTIVITIES OF DAILY LIVING (ADL)

Activities of daily living include getting into cars, unpacking groceries, picking up young children and performing general yard work and typical chores around the house. The stretching program for ADL should focus on the areas that are of most concern from an injury and pain perspective. The neck, upper back, lower back and muscles around the knee should be the main focus.

ACTIVITIES OF DAILY LIVING (ADL) STRETCHES
Upper Trapezius, *page 56*
Lateral Neck Stretch, *page 57*
Neck Flexion Stretch, *page 58*
The Zipper, *page 60*
Seated Shoulder External Rotation, *page 62*
Chest Stretch (with Anchor Position), *page 67*
Lying Wrist/Forearm Stretch (Flexor Focus), *page 69*
Lying Wrist/Forearm Stretch (Extensor Focus), *page 70*
Seated Calf Stretch (Gastrocnemius), *page 72*
Seated Calf Stretch (Soleus), *page 74*
IT Band Stretch, *page 76*
Kneeling Hip Flexor Stretch, *page 81*
Introductory Hip Stretch, *page 86*
Sit & Reach, *page 93*
Lying Hamstring (Straight Leg), *page 96*
BEGINNER: 5 reps INTERMEDIATE: 10 reps ADVANCED: 15 reps

DESK JOB

Individuals who sit at a desk for 6–10 hours per day have specific muscle imbalances, flexibility issues and muscle tightness that result from poor posture and the requirement to maintain certain positions in a static position for many hours at a time. Their stretching program should focus on the neck, upper back, shoulders, wrists and hip flexors.

DESK JOB STRETCHES
Upper Trapezius, *page 56*
Lateral Neck Stretch, *page 57*
Neck Flexion Stretch, *page 58*
The Zipper, *page 60*
Seated Shoulder External Rotation, *page 62*
Chest Stretch, *page 65*
Lying Wrist/Forearm Stretch (Flexor Focus), *page 69*
Lying Wrist/Forearm Stretch (Extensor Focus), *page 70*
Seated Calf Stretch (Gastrocnemius), *page 72*
Seated Calf Stretch (Soleus), *page 74*
Introductory Hip Stretch, *page 86*
Sit & Reach, *page 93*
Lying Hamstring (Bent Leg), *page 97*
BEGINNER: 5 reps INTERMEDIATE: 10 reps ADVANCED: 15 reps

GARDENING

Individuals who garden on a regular basis are prone to lower back, knee and upper-body posture challenges. Their stretching program should focus on increasing range of motion throughout the lower back, hamstrings and upper-back area.

GARDENING STRETCHES
Lateral Neck Stretch, *page 57*
Neck Flexion Stretch, *page 58*
Lying Cross-Body Stretch, *page 64*
Seated Shoulder External Rotation, *page 62*
Chest Stretch, *page 65*
Lying Wrist/Forearm Stretch (Flexor Focus), *page 69*
Lying Wrist/Forearm Stretch (Extensor Focus), *page 70*
Seated Calf Stretch (Gastrocnemius), *page 72*
Seated Calf Stretch (Soleus), *page 74*
Figure-4 Stretch, *page 87*
Kneeling Hip Flexor Stretch, *page 81*
Introductory Hip Stretch, *page 86*
Standing Lower-Back Stretch, *page 92*
Lying Wiper Stretch (Lateral Flexion), *page 95*
Lying Hamstring (Bent Leg), *page 97*
BEGINNER: 5 reps INTERMEDIATE: 10 reps ADVANCED: 15 reps

SHOULDER PROGRAM

Many individuals suffer from shoulder discomfort, tightness or poor posture. This stretching program provides specific stretches to help improve shoulder range of motion throughout the major movements required during most activities.

SHOULDER PROGRAM STRETCHES
Upper Trapezius, *page 56*
Lateral Neck Stretch, *page 57*
Neck Flexion Stretch, *page 58*
Overhead Backward Stretch, *page 59*
The Zipper, *page 60*
Chest Stretch (with Anchor Position), *page 67*
Seated Shoulder External Rotation, *page 62*
Lying Sleeper Stretch (Internal Rotation), *page 63*
Lying Cross-Body Stretch, *page 64*
Chest Stretch, *page 65*
Advanced Chest Stretch, *page 66*
Triceps Stretch, *page 68*
BEGINNER: 5 reps INTERMEDIATE: 10 reps ADVANCED: 15 reps

LOWER-BACK PROGRAM

Many individuals suffer from lower-back discomfort and tightness. This stretching program provides specific stretches to help improve lower-back range of motion throughout the major movements required during most activities.

LOWER-BACK PROGRAM STRETCHES
Seated Calf Stretch (Gastrocnemius), *page 72*
Seated Calf Stretch (Soleus), *page 74*
Lying Calf Stretch (Gastrocnemius), *page 73*
Lying Calf Stretch (Soleus), *page 75*
IT Band Stretch, *page 76*
Kneeling Hip Flexor Stretch, *page 81*
Hip External Rotation, *page 82*
Hip Internal Rotation, *page 83*
Figure-4 Stretch, *page 87*
Pretzel Mermaid Stretch, *page 90*
Lying Spinal Rotation, *page 91*
Standing Lower-Back Stretch, *page 92*
Sit & Reach, *page 93*
Scorpion Stretch, *page 94*
Lying Hamstring (Straight Leg), *page 96*
Lying Wiper Stretch (Lateral Flexion), *page 95*
Standing Squat, *page 99*
Standing Swan Dive, *page 101*
BEGINNER: 5 reps INTERMEDIATE: 10 reps ADVANCED: 15 reps

KNEE PROGRAM

Many individuals suffer from knee pain and discomfort. This program provides specific stretches to help improve muscle and joint range of motion around the knee, including the hamstrings, quadriceps and calf muscles.

KNEE PROGRAM STRETCHES
Seated Calf Stretch (Gastrocnemius), *page 72*
Seated Calf Stretch (Soleus), *page 74*
Lying Calf Stretch (Gastrocnemius), *page 73*
Lying Calf Stretch (Soleus), *page 75*
IT Band Stretch, *page 76*
Kneeling Hip Flexor Stretch, *page 81*
Hip External Rotation, *page 82*
Hip Internal Rotation, *page 83*
Pretzel Mermaid Stretch, *page 90*
Lying Spinal Rotation, *page 91*
Standing Squat, *page 99*
Kneeling Quad Stretch, *page 104*
BEGINNER: 5 reps INTERMEDIATE: 10 reps ADVANCED: 15 reps

HIP PROGRAM

Many individuals suffer from hip discomfort and tightness. The program should provide specific stretches to help improve entire hip range of motion, including internal and external hip movement, hamstring range of motion and hip flexors.

HIP PROGRAM STRETCHES
Lying Quad Stretch, *page 77*
IT Band Stretch, *page 76*
Side-Lying Hip Flexor Stretch, *page 80*
Kneeling Hip Flexor Stretch, *page 81*
Hip External Rotation, *page 82*
Hip Internal Rotation, *page 83*
Facedown Hip Internal Rotation, *page 84*
Facedown Hip External Rotation, *page 85*
Introductory Hip Stretch, *page 86*
Figure-4 Stretch, *page 87*
Frog Stretch, *page 89*
Pretzel Mermaid Stretch, *page 90*
BEGINNER: 5 reps INTERMEDIATE: 10 reps ADVANCED: 15 reps

50+ PROGRAM

As we age, it's common that good posture decreases and certain muscle groups start to tighten and negatively influence posture and function. The stretching program should specifically focus on improving range of motion in the major muscles that typically cause the biggest negative influence on posture: hamstrings, hip flexors, calves and upper back.

50+ PROGRAM STRETCHES
Upper Trapezius, *page 56*
Lateral Neck Stretch, *page 57*
Neck Flexion Stretch, *page 58*
The Zipper, *page 60*
Seated Shoulder External Rotation, *page 62*
Chest Stretch, *page 65*
Lying Wrist/Forearm Stretch (Flexor Focus), *page 69*
Lying Calf Stretch (Gastrocnemius), *page 73*
Lying Calf Stretch (Soleus), *page 75*
Standing Squat, *page 99*
Introductory Hip Stretch, *page 86*
Sit & Reach, *page 93*
Lying Hamstring (Bent Leg), *page 97*
BEGINNER: 5 reps INTERMEDIATE: 10 reps ADVANCED: 15 reps

BASEBALL/SOFTBALL

Baseball and softball are sports that involve high levels of rotational strength and flexibility. Hitting the ball requires an effective kinetic chain transfer from the ground up through the lower body and the core and out through the arms into the bat, which allows for powerful ball contact. Stretching exercises should focus on rotational movements and the shoulder, especially for pitchers.

BASEBALL/SOFTBALL STRETCHES
Lateral Neck Stretch, *page 57*
The Zipper, *page 60*
Lying Shoulder External Rotation, *page 61*
Lying Sleeper Stretch (Internal Rotation), *page 63*
Lying Cross-Body Stretch, *page 64*
Advanced Chest Stretch, *page 66*
Triceps Stretch, *page 68*
IT Band Stretch, *page 76*
Advanced Quad Stretch, *page 79*
Side-Lying Hip Flexor Stretch, *page 80*
Facedown Hip Internal Rotation, *page 84*
Facedown Hip External Rotation, *page 85*
Standing Figure-4 Stretch, *page 88*
Lying Spinal Rotation, *page 91*
Standing Lunge & Rotation, *page 102*
Lying Hamstring (Straight Leg), *page 96*
BEGINNER: 5 reps INTERMEDIATE: 10 reps ADVANCED: 15 reps

BASKETBALL

Basketball places a major emphasis on acceleration, change of direction and jumping ability. Due to the sport's many stop-and-start movements, a stretching program needs to focus on having appropriate range of motion in the movements needed for basketball. Therefore, stretching of the muscles involved in the lower body, hips, back and core is important.

BASKETBALL STRETCHES
Lying Sleeper Stretch (Internal Rotation), *page 63*
Lying Cross-Body Stretch, *page 64*
Advanced Chest Stretch, *page 66*
Triceps Stretch, *page 68*
Advanced Wrist/Forearm Stretch, *page 71*
Seated Calf Stretch (Gastrocnemius), *page 72*
Seated Calf Stretch (Soleus), *page 74*
IT Band Stretch, *page 76*
Advanced Quad Stretch, *page 79*
Kneeling Hip Flexor Stretch, *page 81*
Facedown Hip Internal Rotation, *page 84*
Facedown Hip External Rotation, *page 85*
Standing Figure-4 Stretch, *page 88*
Lying Spinal Rotation, *page 91*
Standing Lower-Back Stretch, *page 92*
Scorpion Stretch, *page 94*
Lying Hamstring (Straight Leg), *page 96*
BEGINNER: 5 reps INTERMEDIATE: 10 reps ADVANCED: 15 reps

BODYBUILDING

Bodybuilding emphasizes size, thickness, symmetry and low body fat. The stretching exercises should allow for you to go through a greater range of motion during the resistance training exercises, thereby enabling you to recruit greater ranges of muscle fibers and helping to increase gains. Also, reducing any muscle imbalances may help lower the injury risk. The exercises should include all the muscles of the body, with specific emphasis on any imbalances or lagging muscle groups.

BODYBUILDING STRETCHES
Lateral Neck Stretch, *page 57*
Lying Shoulder External Rotation, *page 61*
Lying Cross-Body Stretch, *page 64*
Advanced Chest Stretch, *page 66*
Triceps Stretch, *page 68*
Advanced Wrist/Forearm Stretch, *page 71*
Seated Calf Stretch (Gastrocnemius), *page 72*
Seated Calf Stretch (Soleus), *page 74*
Lying Quad Stretch, *page 77*
Side-Lying Hip Flexor Stretch, *page 80*
Facedown Hip Internal Rotation, *page 84*
Facedown Hip External Rotation, *page 85*
Figure-4 Stretch, *page 87*
Sit & Reach, *page 93*
Standing Sumo Squat, *page 100*
Lying Hamstring (Bent Leg), *page 97*
BEGINNER: 5 reps INTERMEDIATE: 10 reps ADVANCED: 15 reps

CYCLING

Cycling is a lower-body-focused activity that requires strength in the quadriceps, hamstrings and calf muscles. The core needs to be strong to help with transition of force through the lower body into the pedals. Hip flexor and hamstring flexibility is vital for efficient pedal cadence and efficiency of movement throughout each pedal cycle. Therefore, the focus of stretching programs should be on improving range of motion of lower-body muscles (quadriceps, hamstrings, calf muscles) and muscles of the upper back to help with overall general posture, which over time can help in the reduction of injuries.

CYCLING STRETCHES
Seated Calf Stretch (Gastrocnemius), *page 72*
Seated Calf Stretch (Soleus), *page 74*
Lying Calf Stretch (Gastrocnemius), *page 73*
Lying Calf Stretch (Soleus), *page 75*
IT Band Stretch, *page 76*
Side-Lying Hip Flexor Stretch, *page 80*
Kneeling Hip Flexor Stretch, *page 81*
Hip External Rotation, *page 82*
Hip Internal Rotation, *page 83*
Pretzel Mermaid Stretch, *page 90*
Sit & Reach, *page 93*
Lying Hamstring (Bent Leg), *page 97*
Standing Squat, *page 99*
Kneeling Quad Stretch, *page 104*
BEGINNER: 5 reps INTERMEDIATE: 10 reps ADVANCED: 15 reps

FOOTBALL, AUSTRALIAN RULES

In Australian Rules Football, large distances must be covered in short amounts of time. Maximal-velocity sprinting is common. Therefore, it's important to improve hamstring and lower-back range of motion. Upper-body range of motion is also important due to the need to catch the ball in unusual positions.

FOOTBALL, AUSTRALIAN RULES STRETCHES
The Zipper, *page 60*
Lying Sleeper Stretch (Internal Rotation), *page 63*
Advanced Chest Stretch, *page 66*
Triceps Stretch, *page 68*
Advanced Wrist/Forearm Stretch, *page 71*
Seated Calf Stretch (Gastrocnemius), *page 72*
Seated Calf Stretch (Soleus), *page 74*
IT Band Stretch, *page 76*
Side-Lying Hip Flexor Stretch, *page 80*
Kneeling Hip Flexor Stretch, *page 81*
Facedown Hip Internal Rotation, *page 84*
Facedown Hip External Rotation, *page 85*
Standing Figure-4 Stretch, *page 88*
Pretzel Mermaid Stretch, *page 90*
Frog Stretch, *page 89*
Lying Spinal Rotation, *page 91*
Standing Lower-Back Stretch, *page 92*
Scorpion Stretch, *page 94*
Lying Hamstring (Straight Leg), *page 96*
BEGINNER: 5 reps INTERMEDIATE: 10 reps ADVANCED: 15 reps

FOOTBALL, SKILL POSITIONS

Skill positions such as running backs, wide receivers and cornerbacks require explosive acceleration with rapid change of direction and deceleration abilities. As hip flexor, hamstring and hip range of motion are vital to improve speed and reduce the likelihood of the most common injuries to skill position players, these muscles need to be the focus of their stretching program.

FOOTBALL, SKILL POSITION STRETCHES
Lying Sleeper Stretch (Internal Rotation), *page 63*
Lying Cross-Body Stretch, *page 64*
Advanced Chest Stretch, *page 66*
Triceps Stretch, *page 68*
Advanced Wrist/Forearm Stretch, *page 71*
Seated Calf Stretch (Gastrocnemius), *page 72*
Seated Calf Stretch (Soleus), *page 74*
IT Band Stretch, *page 76*
Kneeling Quad Stretch, *page 104*
Side-Lying Hip Flexor Stretch, *page 80*
Kneeling Hip Flexor Stretch, *page 81*
Hip External Rotation, *page 82*
Hip Internal Rotation, *page 83*
Standing Figure-4 Stretch, *page 88*
Pretzel Mermaid Stretch, *page 90*
Standing Wiper Stretch (Lateral Flexion), *page 103*
Lying Spinal Rotation, *page 91*
Standing Lower-Back Stretch, *page 92*
Scorpion Stretch, *page 94*
Lying Hamstring (Straight Leg), *page 96*
BEGINNER: 5 reps INTERMEDIATE: 10 reps ADVANCED: 15 reps

FOOTBALL, LINEMAN

The line positions in football require explosive power, predominantly in a linear direction, but there's also a need for quick lateral movements. Good range of motion, especially in the wrists and forearm, are a focus, as well as in the hip flexors and hamstrings to help with acceleration and lower-body power production.

FOOTBALL, LINEMAN STRETCHES
Lateral Neck Stretch, *page 57*
Neck Flexion Stretch, *page 58*
The Zipper, *page 60*
Lying Shoulder External Rotation, *page 61*
Chest Stretch (with Anchor Position), *page 67*
Lying Cross-Body Stretch, *page 64*
Advanced Chest Stretch, *page 66*
Triceps Stretch, *page 68*
Lying Wrist/Forearm Stretch (Flexor Focus), *page 69*
Lying Wrist/Forearm Stretch (Extensor Focus), *page 70*
Advanced Wrist/Forearm Stretch, *page 71*
IT Band Stretch, *page 76*
Lying Quad Stretch, *page 77*
Side-Lying Hip Flexor Stretch, *page 80*
Facedown Hip Internal Rotation, *page 84*
Facedown Hip External Rotation, *page 85*
Figure-4 Stretch, *page 87*
Lying Spinal Rotation, *page 91*
Standing Lunge & Rotation, *page 102*
Lying Hamstring (Bent Leg), *page 97*
BEGINNER: 5 reps INTERMEDIATE: 10 reps ADVANCED: 15 reps

GOLF

Golf requires very large rotational forces and single-effort power movements. Dynamic range of motion at the trunk, hips, core and shoulder girdle are vital to improved performance and reduction in injury. Stretching programs for golf need to focus heavily on rotation in both the upper and lower body. Increasing range and limiting imbalances are important for success.

GOLF STRETCHES
Lateral Neck Stretch, *page 57*
The Zipper, *page 60*
Lying Shoulder External Rotation, *page 61*
Advanced Chest Stretch, *page 66*
Lying Cross-Body Stretch, *page 64*
Chest Stretch (with Anchor Position), *page 67*
Lying Wrist/Forearm Stretch (Flexor Focus), *page 69*
Lying Wrist/Forearm Stretch (Extensor Focus), *page 70*
Advanced Wrist/Forearm Stretch, *page 71*
IT Band Stretch, *page 76*
Lying Calf Stretch (Soleus), *page 75*
Lying Calf Stretch (Gastrocnemius), *page 73*
Kneeling Quad Stretch, *page 104*
Side-Lying Hip Flexor Stretch, *page 80*
Facedown Hip Internal Rotation, *page 84*
Facedown Hip External Rotation, *page 85*
Figure-4 Stretch, *page 87*
Frog Stretch, *page 89*
Pretzel Mermaid Stretch, *page 90*
Lying Spinal Rotation, *page 91*
Standing Lunge & Rotation, *page 102*
Lying Hamstring (Straight Leg), *page 96*
BEGINNER: 5 reps INTERMEDIATE: 10 reps ADVANCED: 15 reps

HOCKEY

Hockey (both on ice and on in-line skates) places a large emphasis on the core and lower-body strength, power and range of motion. The ability to change direction quickly and produce explosive lateral movements are also paramount to success. Stretching for hockey requires focus on the hips and lower body, especially in lateral movements.

HOCKEY STRETCHES
Lateral Neck Stretch, *page 57*
Neck Flexion Stretch, *page 58*
Chest Stretch, *page 65*
Lying Wrist/Forearm Stretch (Flexor Focus), *page 69*
Lying Wrist/Forearm Stretch (Extensor Focus), *page 70*
Advanced Wrist/Forearm Stretch, *page 71*
Side-Lying Quad Stretch, *page 78*
IT Band Stretch, *page 76*
Side-Lying Hip Flexor Stretch, *page 80*
Kneeling Hip Flexor Stretch, *page 81*
Hip External Rotation, *page 82*
Hip Internal Rotation, *page 83*
Facedown Hip Internal Rotation, *page 84*
Facedown Hip External Rotation, *page 85*
Introductory Hip Stretch, *page 86*
Figure-4 Stretch, *page 87*
Frog Stretch, *page 89*
Pretzel Mermaid Stretch, *page 90*
BEGINNER: 5 reps INTERMEDIATE: 10 reps ADVANCED: 15 reps

LACROSSE

Lacrosse athletes require a combination of upper body, lower body and core strength in all planes of motion due to the simultaneous use of upper and lower body for running, catching and throwing. The stretching program needs to be a good overall program targeting the upper and lower body.

LACROSSE STRETCHES
Lateral Neck Stretch, *page 57*
The Zipper, *page 60*
Lying Shoulder External Rotation, *page 61*
Standing Wiper Stretch (Lateral Flexion), *page 103*
Chest Stretch, *page 65*
Triceps Stretch, *page 68*
Lying Wrist/Forearm Stretch (Flexor Focus), *page 69*
Lying Wrist/Forearm Stretch (Extensor Focus), *page 70*
Lying Calf Stretch (Soleus), *page 75*
Lying Calf Stretch (Gastrocnemius), *page 73*
Kneeling Quad Stretch, *page 104*
Side-Lying Hip Flexor Stretch, *page 80*
Facedown Hip Internal Rotation, *page 84*
Facedown Hip External Rotation, *page 85*
Figure-4 Stretch, *page 87*
Frog Stretch, *page 89*
Lying Spinal Rotation, *page 91*
Lying Wiper Stretch (Lateral Flexion), *page 95*
Lying Hamstring (Straight Leg), *page 96*
BEGINNER: 5 reps INTERMEDIATE: 10 reps ADVANCED: 15 reps

RACQUETBALL/SQUASH

Both squash and racquetball have similar physical requirements and need explosive lower-body movements in multiple directions. They also require kinetic chain energy transfer through the ground up and into the strokes. The utilization of rotational strength and range of motion is paramount to success and these components need to be incorporated in the stretching program. It's also important to focus on the shoulder, elbow and wrist of the athlete due to the requirements of swinging the racquet and hitting the ball.

RACQUETBALL/SQUASH STRETCHES
Lateral Neck Stretch, *page 57*
The Zipper, *page 60*
Lying Sleeper Stretch (Internal Rotation), *page 63*
Lying Cross-Body Stretch, *page 64*
Advanced Chest Stretch, *page 66*
Triceps Stretch, *page 68*
Advanced Wrist/Forearm Stretch, *page 71*
Lying Calf Stretch (Gastrocnemius), *page 73*
Lying Calf Stretch (Soleus), *page 75*
IT Band Stretch, *page 76*
Advanced Quad Stretch, *page 79*
Side-Lying Hip Flexor Stretch, *page 80*
Facedown Hip Internal Rotation, *page 84*
Facedown Hip External Rotation, *page 85*
Standing Figure-4 Stretch, *page 88*
Frog Stretch, *page 89*
Lying Spinal Rotation, *page 91*
Standing Lower-Back Stretch, *page 92*
Lying Popliteus, *page 98*
Lying Hamstring (Straight Leg), *page 96*
BEGINNER: 5 reps INTERMEDIATE: 10 reps ADVANCED: 15 reps

RUGBY

Rugby is a sport that requires a combination of power, strength, agility, speed and endurance. Therefore, stretching programs for rugby require movements in all planes of motion. However, a greater emphasis should be placed on the lower back and lower body.

RUGBY STRETCHES
Lateral Neck Stretch, *page 57*
Neck Flexion Stretch, *page 58*
Lying Sleeper Stretch (Internal Rotation), *page 63*
Lying Cross-Body Stretch, *page 64*
Advanced Chest Stretch, *page 66*
Triceps Stretch, *page 68*
Advanced Wrist/Forearm Stretch, *page 71*
Seated Calf Stretch (Gastrocnemius), *page 72*
Seated Calf Stretch (Soleus), *page 74*
IT Band Stretch, *page 76*
Kneeling Quad Stretch, *page 104*
Side-Lying Hip Flexor Stretch, *page 80*
Kneeling Hip Flexor Stretch, *page 81*
Facedown Hip Internal Rotation, *page 84*
Facedown Hip External Rotation, *page 85*
Pretzel Mermaid Stretch, *page 90*
Frog Stretch, *page 89*
Lying Spinal Rotation, *page 91*
Standing Lower-Back Stretch, *page 92*
Scorpion Stretch, *page 94*
Lying Hamstring (Straight Leg), *page 96*
BEGINNER: 5 reps INTERMEDIATE: 10 reps ADVANCED: 15 reps

SNOWBOARDING & SKIING

Skiing emphasizes linear acceleration with some lateral movement. Snowboarding requires stability and balance, as well as very good range of motion. Stretching programs for snowboarding and skiing should focus on linear and lateral planes, as well as the hips and lower body, for improved overall physical performance.

SNOWBOARDING & SKIING STRETCHES
Seated Calf Stretch (Gastrocnemius), *page 72*
Seated Calf Stretch (Soleus), *page 74*
Lying Calf Stretch (Gastrocnemius), *page 73*
Lying Calf Stretch (Soleus), *page 75*
IT Band Stretch, *page 76*
Kneeling Hip Flexor Stretch, *page 81*
Hip External Rotation, *page 82*
Side-Lying Hip Flexor Stretch, *page 80*
Kneeling Hip Flexor Stretch, *page 81*
Hip External Rotation, *page 82*
Hip Internal Rotation, *page 83*
Facedown Hip Internal Rotation, *page 84*
Facedown Hip External Rotation, *page 85*
Figure-4 Stretch, *page 87*
Frog Stretch, *page 89*
Pretzel Mermaid Stretch, *page 90*
Lying Hamstring (Bent Leg), *page 97*
BEGINNER: 5 reps INTERMEDIATE: 10 reps ADVANCED: 15 reps

SOCCER

Soccer is a sport that requires multi-directional movement through all planes of motion. The stretching program should focus on the hips and lower body, with emphasis on the lower back, hamstrings, hip flexors and calf muscles.

SOCCER STRETCHES
Lateral Neck Stretch, *page 57*
Neck Flexion Stretch, *page 58*
Triceps Stretch, *page 68*
Advanced Wrist/Forearm Stretch, *page 71*
Seated Calf Stretch (Gastrocnemius), *page 72*
Seated Calf Stretch (Soleus), *page 74*
IT Band Stretch, *page 76*
Kneeling Quad Stretch, *page 104*
Side-Lying Hip Flexor Stretch, *page 80*
Kneeling Hip Flexor Stretch, *page 81*
Facedown Hip Internal Rotation, *page 84*
Facedown Hip External Rotation, *page 85*
Standing Figure-4 Stretch, *page 88*
Pretzel Mermaid Stretch, *page 90*
Frog Stretch, *page 89*
Lying Spinal Rotation, *page 91*
Lying Popliteus, *page 98*
Scorpion Stretch, *page 94*
Lying Hamstring (Straight Leg), *page 96*
BEGINNER: 5 reps INTERMEDIATE: 10 reps ADVANCED: 15 reps

SWIMMING

Swimming, both sprint and long distances, requires great range of motion of the upper body, trunk and lower body. However, the stretching program should focus heavily on the upper body around the shoulder area, upper back and chest.

SWIMMING STRETCHES
Lateral Neck Stretch, *page 57*
The Zipper, *page 60*
Lying Shoulder External Rotation, *page 61*
Lying Sleeper Stretch (Internal Rotation), *page 63*
Lying Cross-Body Stretch, *page 64*
Advanced Chest Stretch, *page 66*
Side-Lying Quad Stretch, *page 78*
Side-Lying Hip Flexor Stretch, *page 80*
Facedown Hip Internal Rotation, *page 84*
Facedown Hip External Rotation, *page 85*
Standing Lower-Back Stretch, *page 92*
Lying Spinal Rotation, *page 91*
Lying Wiper Stretch (Lateral Flexion), *page 95*
Lying Hamstring (Bent Leg), *page 97*
BEGINNER: 5 reps INTERMEDIATE: 10 reps ADVANCED: 15 reps

TENNIS

Tennis requires a combination of movements to help with energy transfer from the ground up through the kinetic chain. Movements on the tennis court require multi-directional training so a stretching program for a tennis athlete should focus on shoulder internal range of motion, hips, lower back, hamstrings and hip flexors.

TENNIS STRETCHES
Lateral Neck Stretch, *page 57*
The Zipper, *page 60*
Lying Sleeper Stretch (Internal Rotation), *page 63*
Lying Cross-Body Stretch, *page 64*
Advanced Chest Stretch, *page 66*
Triceps Stretch, *page 68*
Advanced Wrist/Forearm Stretch, *page 71*
Lying Calf Stretch (Gastrocnemius), *page 73*
Lying Calf Stretch (Soleus), *page 75*
IT Band Stretch, *page 76*
Advanced Quad Stretch, *page 79*
Side-Lying Hip Flexor Stretch, *page 80*
Kneeling Hip Flexor Stretch, *page 81*
Facedown Hip Internal Rotation, *page 84*
Facedown Hip External Rotation, *page 85*
Standing Figure-4 Stretch, *page 88*
Frog Stretch, *page 89*
Lying Spinal Rotation, *page 91*
Standing Lower-Back Stretch, *page 92*
Scorpion Stretch, *page 94*
Lying Hamstring (Straight Leg), *page 96*
BEGINNER: 5 reps INTERMEDIATE: 10 reps ADVANCED: 15 reps

RUNNING

Running require a stretching program focused on linear movements with emphasis on trunk and hips and the entire lower body. Hip flexors and hamstrings need to be prioritized.

RUNNING STRETCHES
Seated Calf Stretch (Gastrocnemius), *page 72*
Seated Calf Stretch (Soleus), *page 74*
IT Band Stretch, *page 76*
Kneeling Quad Stretch, *page 104*
Side-Lying Hip Flexor Stretch, *page 80*
Kneeling Hip Flexor Stretch, *page 81*
Facedown Hip Internal Rotation, *page 84*
Facedown Hip External Rotation, *page 85*
Standing Figure-4 Stretch, *page 88*
Pretzel Mermaid Stretch, *page 90*
Frog Stretch, *page 89*
Standing Swan Dive, *page 101*
Standing Lower-Back Stretch, *page 92*
Scorpion Stretch, *page 94*
Lying Hamstring (Bent Leg), *page 97*
BEGINNER: 5 reps INTERMEDIATE: 10 reps ADVANCED: 15 reps

VOLLEYBALL

Volleyball focuses on multi-directional movements and a high percentage of vertical movements. Stretching exercises should focus on lower back, hips and lower body, but the upper body also requires extensive work to help with performance and also reduce injury.

VOLLEYBALL STRETCHES
The Zipper, *page 60*
Lying Sleeper Stretch (Internal Rotation), *page 63*
Lying Cross-Body Stretch, *page 64*
Advanced Chest Stretch, *page 66*
Triceps Stretch, *page 68*
Advanced Wrist/Forearm Stretch, *page 71*
Seated Calf Stretch (Gastrocnemius), *page 72*
Seated Calf Stretch (Soleus), *page 74*
IT Band Stretch, *page 76*
Advanced Quad Stretch, *page 79*
Side-Lying Hip Flexor Stretch, *page 80*
Kneeling Hip Flexor Stretch, *page 81*
Facedown Hip Internal Rotation, *page 84*
Facedown Hip External Rotation, *page 85*
Standing Figure-4 Stretch, *page 88*
Frog Stretch, *page 89*
Lying Spinal Rotation, *page 91*
Standing Lower-Back Stretch, *page 92*
Scorpion Stretch, *page 94*
Lying Hamstring (Straight Leg), *page 96*
BEGINNER: 5 reps INTERMEDIATE: 10 reps ADVANCED: 15 reps

PART 3

The Stretches

Upper Trapezius

Target: Upper trapezius

START: Stand up straight and secure one end of the strap under your right foot. Grasp the other end of the strap with your right hand while keeping your elbow straight by your side.

CONTRACT: While keeping your elbow straight, slightly shrug your right shoulder upward. Do not bend your trunk. Hold for 1–2 seconds.

STRETCH: While gently pulling your head away from your right shoulder to stretch your trapezius, slowly breathe out as you relax your right shoulder downward. Stretch for 2 seconds.

Repeat as needed, then switch sides.

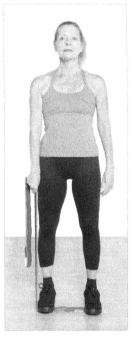

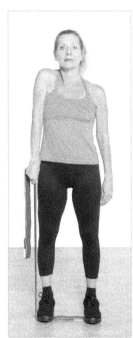

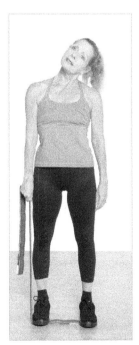

Lateral Neck Stretch

Target: Neck muscles, including the trapezius

Caution: This stretch should be performed in a very slow and controlled manner.

START: Lying on your back on the floor with your legs straight, position the middle of the strap around your head at forehead height. Grasp both ends of the strap with your left hand.

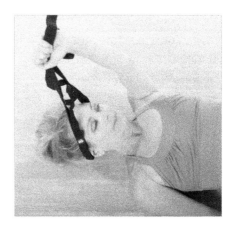

CONTRACT: Slightly push against the strap by tilting your head toward the right while maintaining tension on the strap with your left hand. Hold for 2 seconds.

STRETCH: Slowly breathe out as you relax and very gently and gradually pull the strap toward the left. This should stretch the muscles on the right side of the neck, including the trapezius.

Repeat as needed, then switch sides.

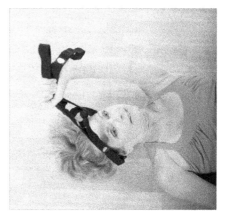

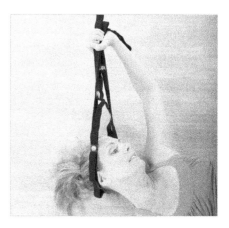

Neck Flexion Stretch

Target: Back of the neck

Caution: This stretch should be performed in a very slow and controlled manner.

START: Lying on your back on the floor with your legs straight, position the strap around your head at forehead height. Grasp both ends of the strap with both hands at eye level, extending your arms directly above your eyes until your arms are straight.

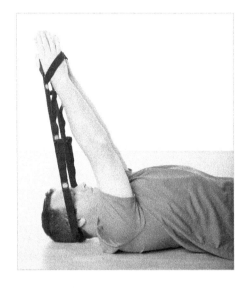

CONTRACT: Slightly push your head down against the strap, toward the ground, while maintaining tension on the strap with your hands. Hold for 1–2 seconds.

STRETCH: Slowly breathe out as you relax and very gently and gradually pull the strap and your head forward. This should stretch the muscles on the back side of the neck. Stretch for 2 seconds.

Repeat as needed, then switch sides.

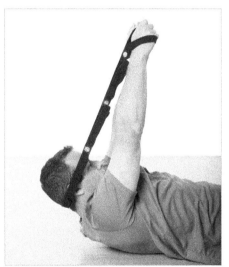

Overhead Backward Stretch

Target: Shoulders, chest, rib cage

START: Standing upright, grasp one end of the strap in each hand. Extend both arms straight above your head with your arms slightly wider than shoulder width.

CONTRACT: While maintaining this starting position, press your arms directly upward by raising your shoulders. Hold for 1–2 seconds.

STRETCH: Breathe out slowly as you move your arms over and behind your head, using the muscles of the upper back to stretch the muscles of the shoulders, chest and rib cage. Hold for 2 seconds.

Return to starting position and repeat as needed.

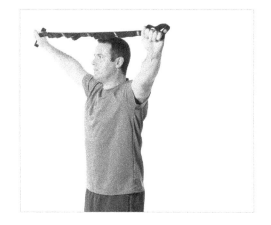

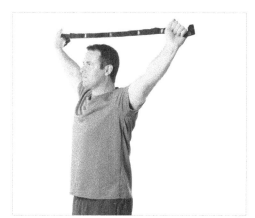

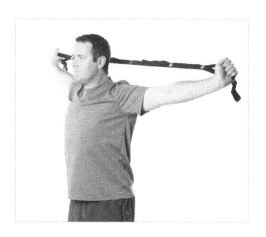

The Zipper

Target: Shoulder

START: Grasp one end of the strap with your left hand behind your lower back. Grasp the other end of the strap with your right hand at head height.

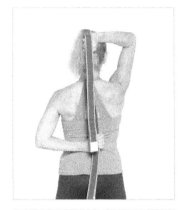

CONTRACT: While maintaining the position of your right elbow at head height, pull down on the strap with your left hand by extending your left elbow. Hold for 2 seconds.

STRETCH: Breathe out slowly as you pull upward with your right arm by extending your right elbow. This movement helps to bring your left hand higher up your lower back, stretching the left shoulder (internal rotation). Stretch for 1–2 seconds.

Repeat as needed, then switch sides.

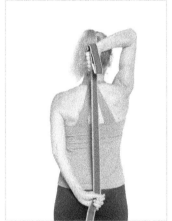

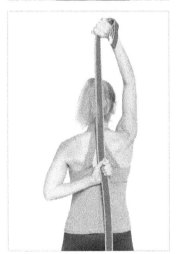

Lying Shoulder External Rotation

Target: Shoulder

START: Lie on your back on a bench, bed or table that can support your weight; keep your eyes staring up at the ceiling. Secure one end of the strap under the bench in line with your head/shoulder region. Squeeze your shoulder blades together and then bend your right elbow 90 degrees. Grasp the other end of the strap with your right hand, palm facing forward.

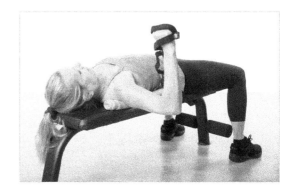

CONTRACT: Pull your right hand upward against the strap. Rotate your right arm internally (toward the middle of your body). During this movement aim to keep your shoulder blades together and elbow bent approximately 90 degrees. Hold for 1–2 seconds.

STRETCH: Slowly breathe out as you allow the strap to gently pull your right shoulder into external rotation (away from your midline), thereby gently stretching the front of your shoulder. Hold for 2 seconds.

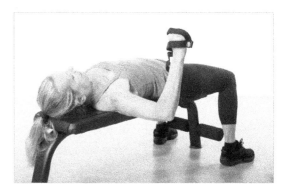

Repeat as needed, then switch sides.

VARIATION: Use a small rolled-up towel to support your upper arm between the back of your arm and the bench. This puts more emphasis on two of the most important muscles of the rotator cuff group: infraspinatus and teres minor.

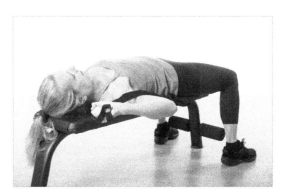

Seated Shoulder External Rotation

Target: Shoulder

START: Sit on a chair or the floor with your back straight and head facing forward. With your right shoulder and elbow at a 90-degree angle, position the middle loop of the strap around your right hand with the strap positioned behind your right forearm/elbow. Grasp the other end with your left hand, keeping the arm in front of your body.

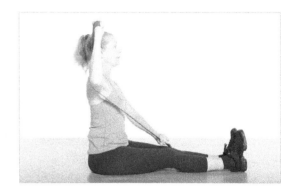

CONTRACT: Slowly push your right hand forward against the strap. Hold for 1–2 seconds.

STRETCH: Slowly pulling the strap forward with your left hand, slowly bring your right hand backward by rotating your shoulder away from your midline. Hold for 2 seconds.

Repeat as needed, then switch sides.

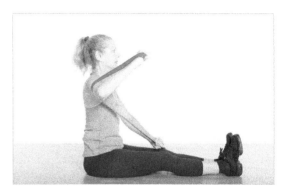

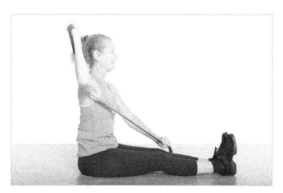

Lying Sleeper Stretch (Internal Rotation)

Target: Shoulder

START: Lie on your right side with your legs straight. Position your right shoulder on the ground and create 90-degree angles at the shoulder and elbow. Position the middle of the strap in your right hand and grasp the ends of the strap with your left hand at around waist level.

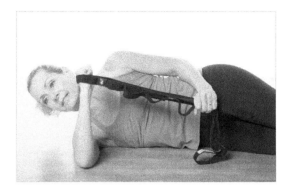

CONTRACT: Holding the strap in your right hand, pull your right hand slowly toward your head by slightly rotating your shoulder away from your midline (externally). Try to keep your shoulder stable and elbow bent approximately 90 degrees. Hold for 1–2 seconds.

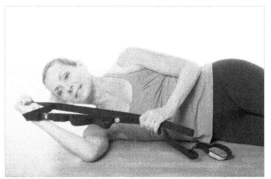

STRETCH: Breathe out as you slowly pull the two ends of the strap with your left hand, bringing your right forearm forward and your wrist toward the floor, thereby gradually stretching the back side of the shoulder. Hold for 2 seconds.

Repeat as needed, then switch sides.

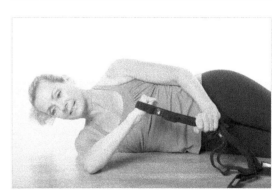

Lying Cross-Body Stretch

Target: Back of the shoulder

START: Lie on your back, pressing your right shoulder blade into the ground. Wrap the middle of the strap around your right hand and grasp both ends of the strap with your left hand. Keep your shoulder blade against the ground while slightly bending your right elbow. Pull slightly away with your left arm to create tension on the strap.

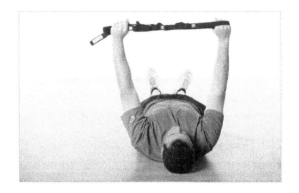

CONTRACT: With your right hand, slowly push against the strap toward the right side of your body, contracting the muscles around your right shoulder, upper back and arm. Hold for 1–2 seconds.

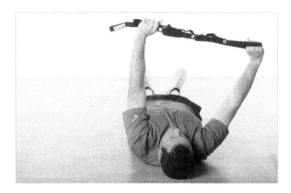

STRETCH: While keeping your right shoulder blade against the ground, breathe out as you slowly pull the strap with your left hand away from the midline of your body toward your left side. This movement stretches the muscles of the back of the shoulder. Hold for 2 seconds.

Repeat as needed, then switch sides.

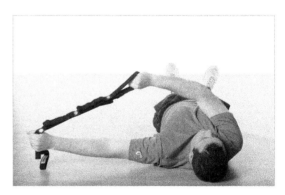

Chest Stretch

Target: Pectoralis major and minor

START: Grasp one end of the strap in each hand. Keeping your elbows straight, extend your arms out to the sides and slightly in front of your body at shoulder height.

CONTRACT: While maintaining tension on the strap, contract your chest muscles by pushing against the strap without any noticeable movement. Hold for 1–2 seconds.

STRETCH: Breathe out as you slowly push your chest forward, moving your arms slightly behind the midline of your body and stretching your chest muscles. Hold for 2 seconds.

Repeat as needed.

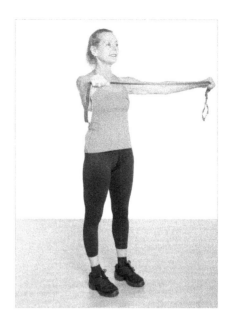

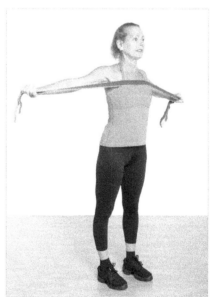

Advanced Chest Stretch

Target: Pectoralis major and minor

This is an advanced stretch because you'll need to coordinate your arms while moving through the exercise, which takes more balance than the basic chest stretch.

START: Grasp one end of the strap in each hand. Keeping your elbows straight, extend your arms out to the sides and slightly above your head in a "Y" position.

CONTRACT: While maintaining tension on the strap, contract your chest muscles while pushing against the strap without any noticeable movement. Hold for 1–2 seconds.

STRETCH: Breathe out as you slowly push your chest forward and slowly lower your arms down behind your head. Stretch for 2 seconds.

To safely get out of the stretch, slowly release the tension on the strap.

Repeat as needed, then switch sides.

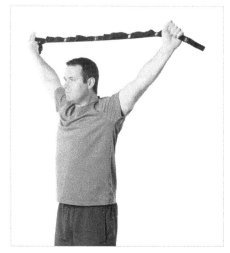

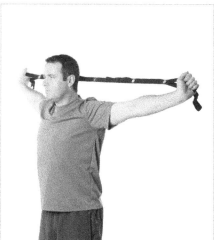

Chest Stretch (with Anchor Position)

Target: Pectoralis major and minor

START: Anchor the middle loop of the strap against an immobile anchor (nail, clip, post, etc.) at or slightly above head height. Stand with your feet together and your body facing away from the anchor, and grasp one end of the strap in each hand. Position both arms straight out to the sides with your hands at shoulder height, making a cross.

CONTRACT: Squeeze your chest muscles and attempt to move your arms forward against the resistance for 1–2 seconds.

STRETCH: Keeping your feet firmly on the ground, breathe out as you slowly allow your upper body to stretch forward, increasing the stretch throughout the chest. If you need to increase the stretch even more, take 1–2 steps farther away from the anchor. Hold for 2 seconds.

Repeat as needed.

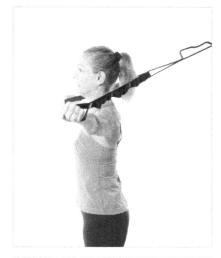

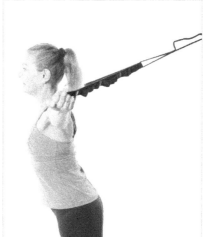

Triceps Stretch

Target: Triceps

START: While standing up straight, grasp one end of the strap with your right hand at head height. Grasp the other end of the strap with your left hand behind your back at the lumbar region (lower back).

CONTRACT: Maintaining the position of your right elbow at head height, pull up on the strap with your right hand by extending your elbow for 1–2 seconds.

STRETCH: Breathe out slowly as you pull down with your left arm, causing your right hand to move slightly down your back by flexing your elbow. This stretches the triceps of your right arm. Hold for 2 seconds.

Repeat as needed, then switch sides.

VARIATION: This can also be performed while sitting in a chair or on the floor.

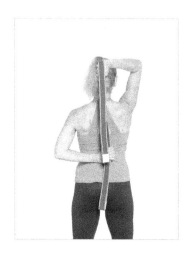

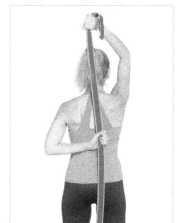

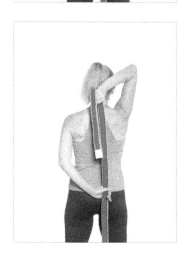

Lying Wrist/Forearm Stretch (Flexor Focus)

Target: Forearm flexors

START: Lie on the floor with your legs straight. Grasp one end of the strap in your left hand (fingers pointing out and bottom of the palm facing upward) and position the other end of the strap around your left foot. While keeping both your arm and leg straight, raise your left leg upward as if stretching your hamstring. This movement creates tension.

CONTRACT: Slowly turn your left wrist downward (fingers pointing out) while simultaneously contracting your forearm for 1–2 seconds.

STRETCH: Breathe out as you slowly lower your leg, increasing the stretch of the wrist flexors. Hold for 2 seconds.

Repeat as needed, then switch sides.

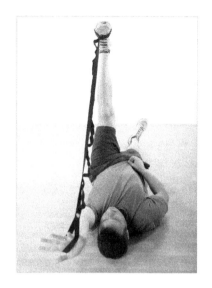

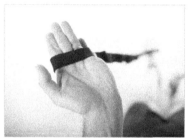

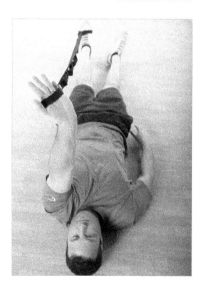

Lying Wrist/Forearm Stretch (Extensor Focus)

Target: Forearm extensors

START: Lie on the floor with your legs straight. Grasp one end of the strap with your left hand (fingers pointing upward and bottom of the palm facing inward) and position the other end of the strap around your left foot. While keeping both your arm and leg straight, raise your left leg upward as if stretching your hamstring. This movement creates tension.

CONTRACT: Slowly turn your left wrist downward (fingers toward to the ground) while simultaneously contracting your forearm. Hold for 1–2 seconds.

STRETCH: Breathe out as you slowly lower your leg, which increases the stretch of the wrist extensors. Hold for 2 seconds.

Repeat as needed, then switch sides.

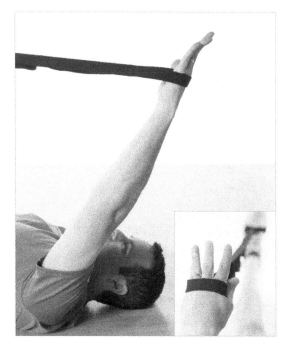

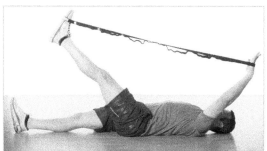

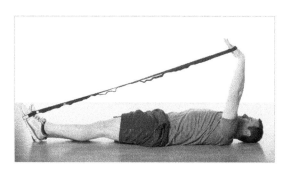

Advanced Wrist/Forearm Stretch

Target: Forearm flexor

This is a more-advanced exercise as you need to position your entire upper body over your wrist and shift your weight away from the anchor. This requires greater upper-body strength and body control to effectively perform the movement.

START: Anchor both ends of the strap around a post or another solid object like the leg of a bed or table. While kneeling on the ground, wrap the middle of the strap around your left wrist/forearm. Position your fingers so they're pointing away from the anchor, and keep your arm straight.

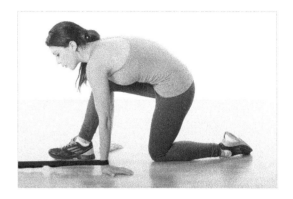

CONTRACT: Keeping your arm straight and forearm roughly perpendicular to the ground, move away from the anchor to ensure that there's enough distance to allow for an isometric contraction of your forearm and wrist. Hold for 1–2 seconds.

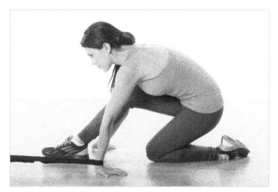

STRETCH: Breathe out as you shift your upper body weight slowly away from the anchor, increasing the stretch through the extensor muscles. Hold for 2 seconds.

Repeat as needed, then switch sides.

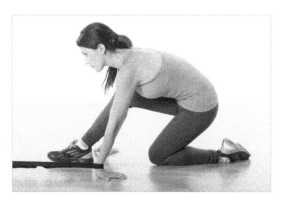

Seated Calf Stretch (Gastrocnemius)

Target: Gastrocnemius

The calf is composed of two main muscles: the gastrocnemius and the soleus. This stretch works the gastrocnemius, the larger calf muscle.

START: Sit on the floor with your legs and back straight. Place the middle of the strap around your left foot and grasp both ends of the strap with both hands at approximately waist level.

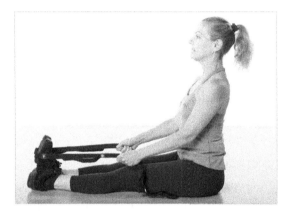

CONTRACT: Keeping your leg straight, slowly push your foot downward against the strap by pointing your toes (plantar flexion). Maintain your hand position and good upper body posture to ensure that tension is maintained on the strap. Hold for 1–2 seconds.

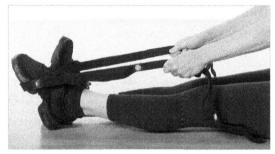

STRETCH: Slowly breathe out as you pull the straps toward your chest, moving your left foot toward you so that you're flexing your foot (dorsiflexion). This increases the range of motion around your ankle and specifically focuses on stretching the gastrocnemius. Hold for 2 seconds.

Repeat as needed, then switch sides.

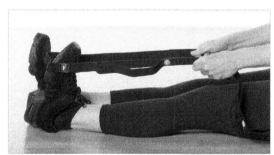

Lying Calf Stretch (Gastrocnemius)

Target: Gastrocnemius

START: Lying on your back, place the middle of the strap around your right foot and grasp both ends of the strap with your hands at approximately waist level. Slowly lift your right leg up, bringing your foot toward your head while keeping your leg straight.

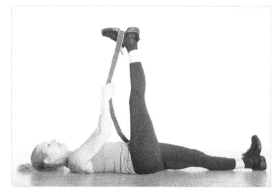

CONTRACT: Keeping your leg straight and maintaining your hand position and good upper body posture, slowly push your foot upward against the strap by pointing your toes (plantar flexion). Hold for 1–2 seconds.

STRETCH: Slowly breathe out as you pull the straps downward toward your chest, which moves your right foot toward you by flexing the foot (dorsiflexion). This increases the range of motion around your ankle and specifically focuses on stretching the gastrocnemius. Hold for 2 seconds.

Repeat as needed, then switch sides.

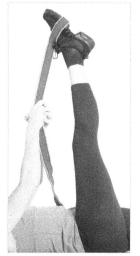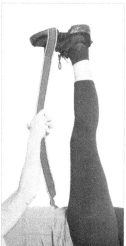

Seated Calf Stretch (Soleus)

Target: Soleus

The calf is composed of two main muscles: the gastrocnemius and the soleus. This stretch works the soleus, the deeper calf muscle.

START: Sit on the floor with your back straight, your right leg extended straight out and your left knee bent approximately 45 degrees. Place the middle of the strap around your left foot and grasp both ends of the strap with your hands at approximately waist level.

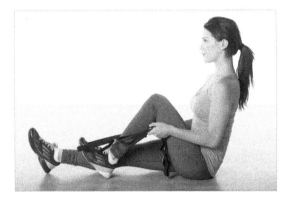

CONTRACT: Maintaining your hand position, good upper body posture and bent knee, slowly push your foot downward by pointing your toes (plantar flexion) against the strap. Hold for 1–2 seconds.

STRETCH: Slowly breathe out as you pull the straps toward your chest, bringing your left foot toward you by flexing the foot (dorsiflexion). Be careful to maintain the bend in the knee to ensure that the soleus muscle is the major focus of the stretch. This increases the range of motion around your ankle. If the knee straightens during the stretch, it shifts the stretch back to more of a gastrocnemius-focused movement. Hold for 2 seconds.

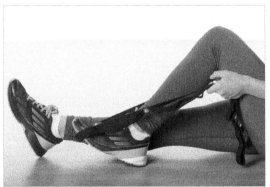

Repeat as needed, then switch sides.

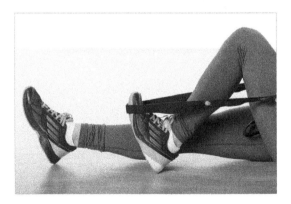

Lying Calf Stretch (Soleus)

Target: Soleus

START: Lie on your back with your right leg straight and your left knee slightly bent. Place the middle of the strap around your left foot and grasp both ends of the strap with your hands at approximately your waist. Bring your left leg toward your chest, maintaining the slight bend in your knee.

CONTRACT: Keeping your right leg straight, maintaining your hand position while lying on the ground and keeping your left knee bent, slowly push your left foot upward against the strap by pointing your toes (plantar flexion). Hold for 1–2 seconds.

STRETCH: Slowly breathe out as you pull the straps toward your chest, moving your left foot toward you by flexing the foot (dorsiflexion). This increases the range of motion around your ankle and specifically focuses on stretching the soleus. Hold for 2 seconds.

Repeat as needed, then switch sides.

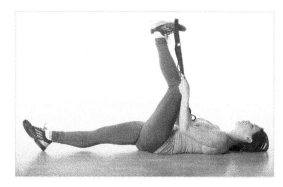

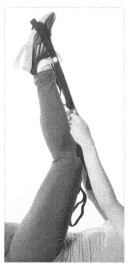
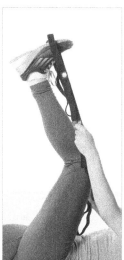

IT Band Stretch

Target: Iliotibial band

START: Lie on your right side with your right hip on the ground and place your right foot in the loop of one end of the strap. Grasp the other end with your hands at waist level and extend your right leg. Bend your left leg and place your left foot in front of your right knee. Slowly lift the right leg 6 to 12 inches off the floor, slightly in front of your midline.

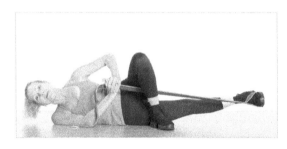

CONTRACT: While keeping your right knee straight and maintaining your hands at waist/chest level, slowly push your right leg down toward the floor against the strap. Hold for 1–2 seconds.

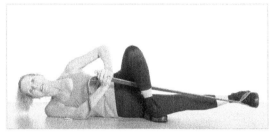

STRETCH: Slowly breathe out as you pull the strap toward your head, lifting your right leg while keeping it straight. Hold for 2 seconds.

Repeat as needed, then switch sides.

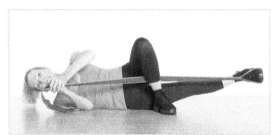

Lying Quad Stretch

Target: Quadriceps

START: Lying facedown with your legs extended along the ground, secure one end of the strap to your left foot and bend your left knee. Grasp the other end of the strap in your left hand over your left shoulder.

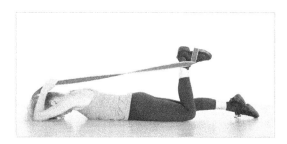

CONTRACT: While maintaining your hand position, slowly push your foot against the strap toward the floor by extending your knee. Hold for 1–2 seconds.

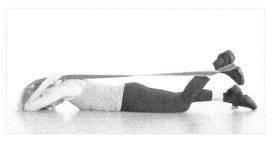

STRETCH: Breathe out as you pull the strap over your left shoulder, stretching your left thigh as your left knee bends, bringing your left foot toward your left buttock. Hold for 1–2 seconds.

Repeat as needed, then switch sides.

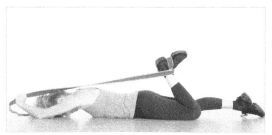

Side-Lying Quad Stretch

Target: Quadriceps

START: Lie on your left side with both legs slightly bent. Secure one end of the strap to your right foot and grasp the other end of the strap in your right hand behind your back. Slowly pull on the strap, causing your right knee to flex, bringing your right foot toward your right hamstring.

CONTRACT: While maintaining your hand position and body posture, slowly push your right foot into the strap by contracting the quadriceps muscles. Hold for 1–2 seconds.

STRETCH: Breathe out as you pull the strap above your right shoulder, stretching your right thigh as you slowly bend your right knee, bringing your right foot toward your right buttock. Hold for 2 seconds.

Repeat as needed, then switch sides.

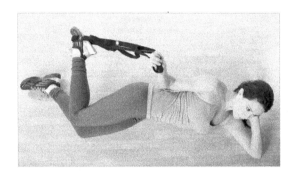

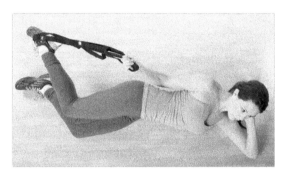

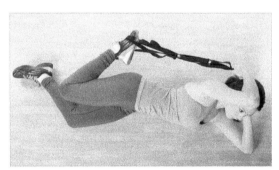

Advanced Quad Stretch

Target: Quadriceps

This is more advanced because it requires balance and coordination of the trunk and upper body, and a base level of flexibility is needed to even get into the starting position.

START: Sit on the floor with the outside of your right hip, thigh and calf on the ground and your right knee bent. Keep your upper body erect, with your back and head in line with each other. Your left hip will be pointing forward. Position the middle of the strap round your left foot and grasp both ends of the strap with your left hand.

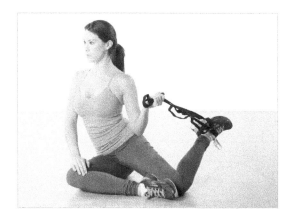

CONTRACT: While maintaining your hand position, slowly push your left foot against the strap, extending your foot away from your body. (You may grab the strap with both hands if necessary.) Hold for 1–2 seconds.

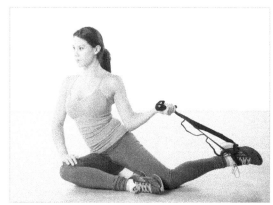

STRETCH: Breathe out as you pull on the strap, bringing your foot closer to your left buttock. Hold for 2 seconds.

Repeat as needed, then switch sides.

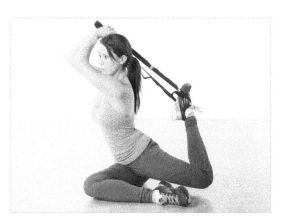

Side-Lying Hip Flexor Stretch

Target: Hip flexors

START: Lie on your left side on the ground with your left knee slightly bent. Place your right foot in the loop of one end of the strap and allow your knee to bend while grasping the other end of the strap with your right hand around waist level.

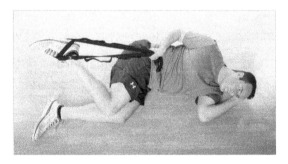

CONTRACT: While keeping the right leg bent, slowly push your hip and thigh forward against the strap (this will be a fairly subtle movement). Maintain the hand position at waist level. Hold for 1–2 seconds.

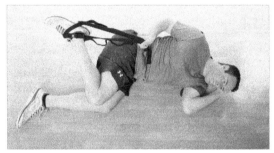

STRETCH: Slowly breathe out as you pull the strap with your right hand in front of your face, pulling your right foot back behind your body, stretching the front of your hip (hip flexors). Hold for 2 seconds.

Repeat as needed, then switch sides.

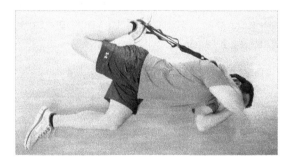

Kneeling Hip Flexor Stretch

Target: Hip flexors

START: Place a stability pad (or a rolled-up towel) on the ground and place your left knee on the pad while your right foot is on the ground in front of you with the knee bent approximately 90 degrees. Place your left foot in the loop of one end of the strap and allow the knee to bend while grasping the other end of the strap at hip level with your left hand.

CONTRACT: While keeping your left leg bent and maintaining your hand position at hip level, slowly push your left foot against the strap and toward the ground by contracting your hip flexors. Hold for 1–2 seconds.

STRETCH: Slowly breathe out as you pull the strap with your left hand over your left shoulder, bringing your left foot up toward your left buttocks, stretching the front of your hip (hip flexors). Hold for 2 seconds.

Repeat as needed, then switch sides.

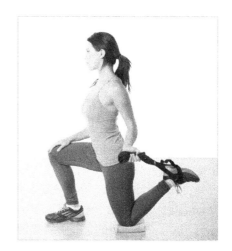

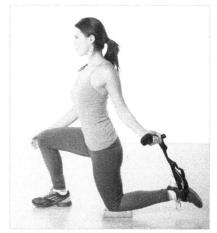

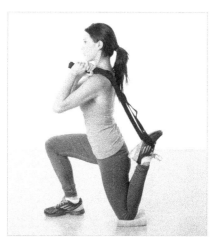

Hip External Rotation

Target: 6 major muscles involved in hip rotation, including piriformis, gemellus superior, obturator externus, and quadratus femoris

START: Lie on your back with your left leg straight and your right hip and knee both bent 90 degrees and your right foot in the air. Secure your right foot into a loop of the strap and grasp the ends of the strap with both hands around stomach level.

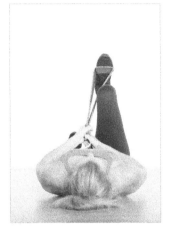

CONTRACT: While maintaining the hand position, slowly push your right leg very slightly to the right against the strap. Keep your right hip at approximately 90 degrees and the lower leg parallel to the floor. Although the muscles are contracting, very little to no movement is occurring at the hip. Hold for 1–2 seconds.

STRETCH: Breathe out as you slowly pull the strap toward your left shoulder, which brings your right foot and lower right leg toward your left hip and your knee across your body, stretching the hip muscles. Hold for 2 seconds.

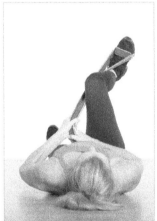

Repeat as needed, then switch sides.

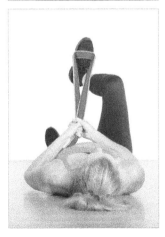

Hip Internal Rotation

Target: 7 major muscles in hip internal rotation, including gluteus medius, gluteus minimus, and tensor fascia latae

START: Lie on your back with your left leg straight and your right hip and knee both bent 90 degrees. Secure your right foot into a loop of the strap and grasp the ends of the strap with both hands around stomach level.

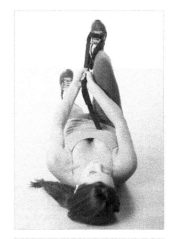

CONTRACT: While maintaining your hand position, slowly push your right leg very slightly to the left against the strap. Keep your hip at approximately 90 degrees and the lower leg parallel to the floor. Although the muscles are contracting, very little to no movement is occurring at the hip. Hold for 1–2 seconds.

STRETCH: Breathe out as you slowly pull the strap slightly away from your body, bringing your right knee across your body and your lower right leg out toward the right, stretching the internal rotator muscles of your hip. Stretch for 2 seconds.

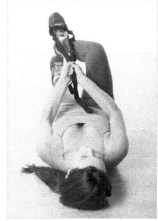

Repeat as needed, then switch sides.

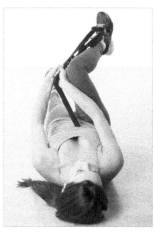

Facedown Hip Internal Rotation

Target: 7 major muscles in hip internal rotation, including gluteus medius, gluteus minimus, and tensor fascia latae

START: Lie on your stomach with your forehead resting on your left forearm on the ground. Bend your right knee approximately 90 degrees. Secure your right foot into a loop of the strap and grasp the ends of the strap with your right hand on the right side of your body.

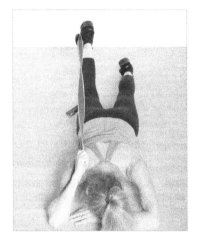

CONTRACT: While maintaining your hand position, slowly push your right leg against the strap, creating an isometric contraction. Keep your hip stable and knee flexed at approximately 90 degrees and your lower leg perpendicular to the floor. Although the muscles are contracting, very little to no movement is occurring at the hip. Hold for 1–2 seconds.

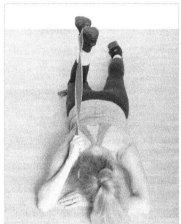

STRETCH: Breathe out as you slowly pull the strap with your right hand slightly away from your body, which brings your right foot/lower right leg slightly outside the line of the right hip, stretching the internal hip rotator muscles. Hold for 2 seconds.

Repeat as needed, then switch sides.

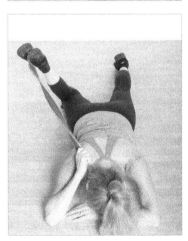

Facedown Hip External Rotation

Target: 6 major muscles involved in hip rotation, including piriformis, gemellus superior, obturator externus, and quadratus femoris

START: Lie on your stomach with your forehead resting on your left forearm on the ground. Bend your right knee approximately 90 degrees. Secure your right foot into a loop of the strap and grasp the ends of the strap with your right hand on the right side of your body.

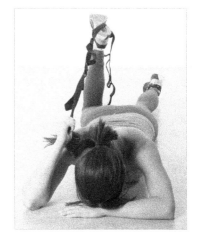

CONTRACT: While maintaining your hand position, slowly push your right leg against the strap, creating an isometric contraction. Keep your hip stable and knee bent and the lower leg perpendicular to the floor. Although the muscles are contracting, very little to no movement is occurring at the hip. Hold for 1–2 seconds.

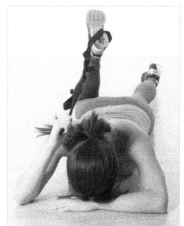

STRETCH: Breathe out as you slowly pull the strap with your right hand slightly toward the midline of your body, bringing your right foot and lower right leg slightly to the inside of the upper right leg, stretching the external hip rotator muscles. Stretch for 2 seconds.

Repeat as needed, then switch sides.

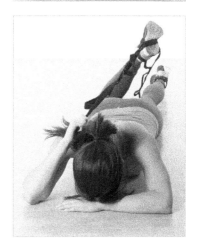

Introductory Hip Stretch

Target: Piriformis

This is considered an introductory stretch because it requires less movement and can be performed by most people, even if they have limited range of motion.

START: Lie on your back with your left knee bent and left foot on the ground. Place the outside of your right foot on your left thigh. Place the middle of the strap around your right knee, and grasp both ends of the strap with your left hand around hip level.

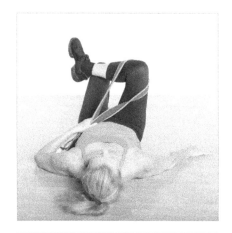

CONTRACT: While maintaining your hand position and keeping your right foot on your left thigh, slowly push your right leg away from your trunk against the strap. Hold for 1–2 seconds.

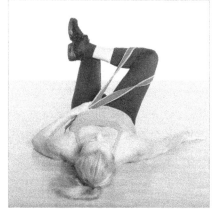

STRETCH: Breathe out as you pull the strap toward your left shoulder, bringing your right leg toward the midline of your body. Hold for 2 seconds.

Repeat as needed, then switch sides.

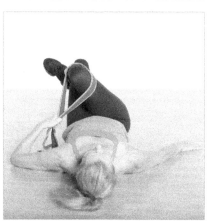

Figure-4 Stretch

Target: Piriformis

START: Lie on your back with your left knee and left hip both bent 90 degrees. Your left toes should be pointing toward the sky with your leg off the ground. Place the outside of your right foot on your left thigh and place the middle of the strap around your left foot, grasping both ends of the strap with both hands around hip level.

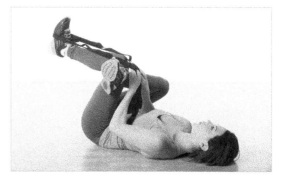

CONTRACT: While maintaining your hand position and keeping your right foot on your left thigh, slowly push your right leg away from your trunk against the strap. Hold for 1–2 seconds.

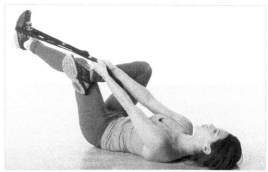

STRETCH: Breathe out as you pull the strap toward your left shoulder, bringing your left leg toward the midline of your body and stretching your right hip. Hold for 2 seconds.

Repeat as needed, then switch sides.

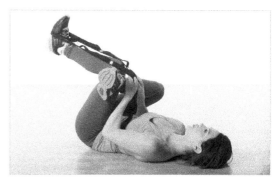

Standing Figure-4 Stretch

Target: Piriformis

START: Anchor the middle loop of the strap against an immobile object (nail, clip, post, etc.) at head height. Standing upright facing the anchor, grasp one end of the strap in each hand. Place the outside of your left foot on your right thigh and slowly bend down, pushing your weight into your right hip, attempting to achieve an approximate 90-degree angle at your left knee.

CONTRACT: Keeping your left foot on your right thigh, slowly push your left leg away from your trunk. Hold for 1–2 seconds.

STRETCH: Breathe out as you sink down, pushing your weight into your left hip while holding the strap at head height, increasing the stretch throughout your left hip. Hold for 2 seconds.

Repeat as needed, then switch sides.

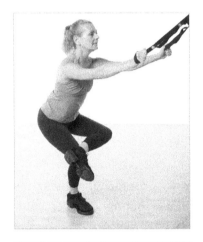

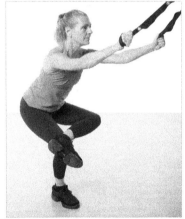

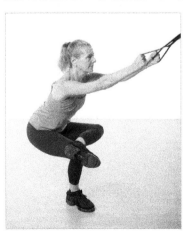

Frog Stretch

Target: Adductors

START: Kneeling on the floor, take your knees apart and put your feet together, forming a diamond with your lower body. Position the strap around both ankles and grasp the end of the strap in your left hand.

CONTRACT: Slowly push your legs into the strap toward the ground. You can place your free hand on the ground for balance. Hold for 1–2 seconds.

STRETCH: Breathe out as you sink down, pushing your weight into the ground while simultaneously pulling on the strap with your left hand to increase the stretch. Hold for 2 seconds.

Repeat as needed.

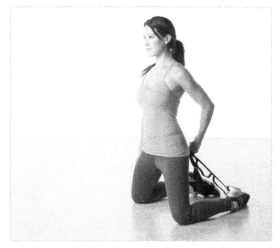

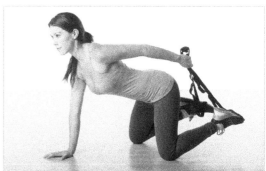

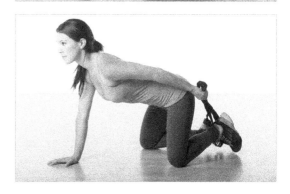

Pretzel Mermaid Stretch

Target: Glutes, hips

START: Lie on your left side with your head on the ground. Reach down and place the middle loop of the strap around your left foot, and grasp both ends of the strap in your right hand. Place your left hand on your right knee.

CONTRACT: Slowly push your left foot into the strap. Hold for 1–2 seconds.

STRETCH: Breathe out and roll your right shoulder blade to the floor as you simultaneously and slowly pull the strap upward, bringing your left foot slightly toward your lower back. Hold for 2 seconds.

Repeat as needed, then switch sides.

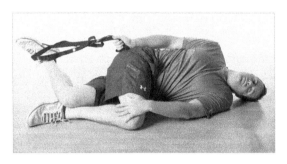

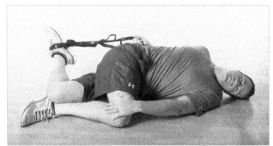

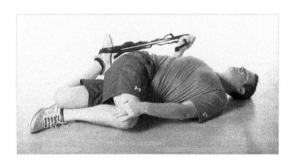

Lying Spinal Rotation

Target: Lower back

START: Lie on your back, bend both knees and bring both feet toward your buttocks while keeping your feet on the floor. Wrap the strap around both thighs and grasp both ends of the strap in your left hand. Position your right arm with your elbow at a 45-degree angle at shoulder level.

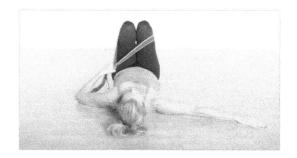

CONTRACT: Slowly contract the muscles of your lower back and hips and push against the strap to your right. Hold for 1–2 seconds.

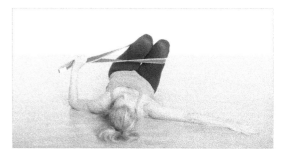

STRETCH: Breathe out as you slowly pull the strap toward your left, dropping your knees toward the ground. This stretches the right side of your lower back and increases spinal rotation range of motion. Stretch for 2 seconds.

Repeat as needed, then switch sides.

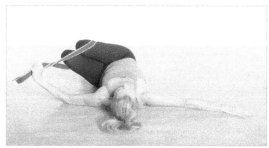

Standing Lower-Back Stretch

Target: Lower back

START: Anchor the middle loop of the strap against an immobile object (nail, clip, post, etc.) above head height. Standing upright facing the anchor, grasp one end of the strap in each hand.

CONTRACT: Slowly bring your hands down toward eye level. Hold for 1–2 seconds.

STRETCH: Breathe out as you squat down while simultaneously raising your hands above your head, stretching out your lower back. Hold for 2 seconds.

Repeat as needed.

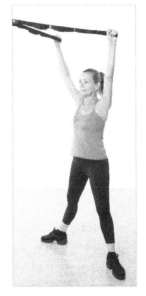

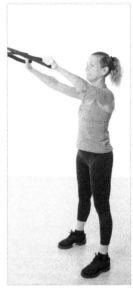

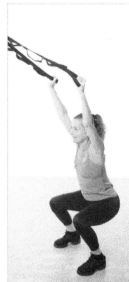

Sit & Reach

Target: Lower back, hamstrings

START: Sit on the floor with your legs extended in front of you while keeping your back straight. Grasp one end of the strap in each hand. Position the middle of the strap around the arches of both feet.

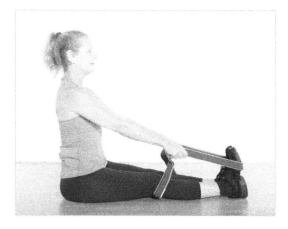

CONTRACT: While holding both ends of the strap, slowly push your legs into the strap by slightly pointing your toes. Hold for 1–2 seconds.

STRETCH: Breathe out as you simultaneously pull the strap toward you with both hands and slowly lean your upper body forward while keeping your lower back straight. This increases the stretch in your lower back and hamstrings. Hold for 2 seconds.

Repeat as needed.

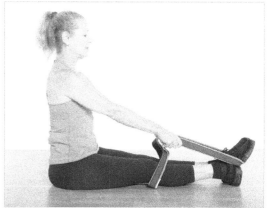

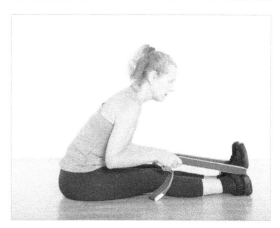

Scorpion Stretch

Target: Lower back, hips

START: Lie on your stomach with your legs straight and together. Place the loop of the strap around your right foot and grasp both ends of the strap in your left hand. Slowly bring your right foot toward your left elbow, positioning your right foot on the outside of your left hip.

CONTRACT: Slowly push your right leg into the strap, slightly pushing your foot away from your body. Hold for 1–2 seconds.

STRETCH: Breathe out as you pull the strap up with your hands and slowly to the left, bringing your right foot closer to your left elbow and stretching your lower back. Hold for 2 seconds.

Repeat as needed, then switch sides.

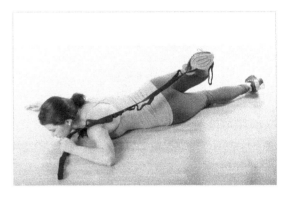

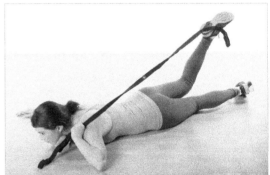

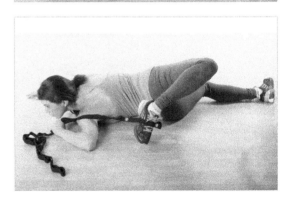

Lying Wiper Stretch (Lateral Flexion)

Target: Obliques, erector spinae, lower back

START: Lie on your back with both arms straight above your head and the middle loop of the strap in the palm of your right hand. Grasp both ends of the strap with your left hand.

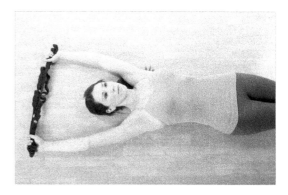

CONTRACT: Slightly move your right hand over your head and toward the midline of the body, increasing the contraction. Hold for 1–2 seconds.

STRETCH: Breathe out as you slowly pull the strap with your left hand to your left side while keeping your right arm straight above your head. The movement should occur from the shift in the muscles on the right side of your core/trunk (lateral flexors). Stretch for 2 seconds.

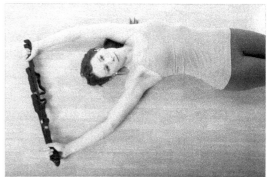

Repeat as needed, then switch sides.

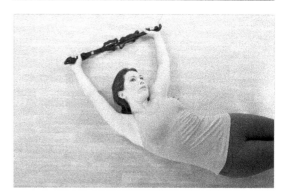

Lying Hamstring (Straight Leg)

Target: Hamstrings

START: Lie on your back with both legs straight. Secure your right foot into a loop of the strap and grasp the ends of the strap with both hands around waist level.

CONTRACT: While keeping your leg straight, slowly pull on the strap to bring your right leg toward your head. Once the leg has reached a stretched position, slowly push your heel away from your body, resulting in a slight contraction. Hold for 1–2 seconds.

STRETCH: Breathe out as you slowly pull the strap with both hands so that your right foot moves toward your head while maintaining a straight leg. Stretch for 2 seconds.

Repeat as needed, then switch sides.

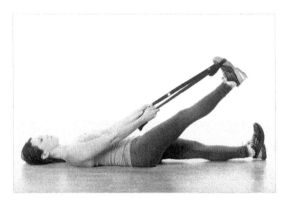

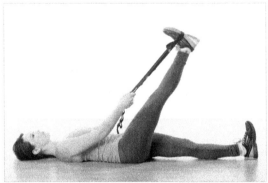

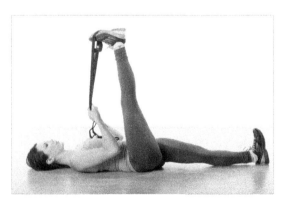

Lying Hamstring (Bent Leg)

Target: Hamstring muscles

START: Lie on your back with your left leg straight and your right leg slightly bent (approximately 75 degrees). Secure your right foot into a loop of the strap and grasp the ends of the strap with both hands around knee level.

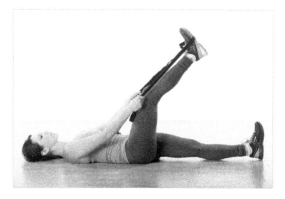

CONTRACT: While maintaining the slight bend in your knee, slowly pull on the strap to bring your right leg toward your head. Once the leg has reached a stretched position, slowly push your heel away from your body, resulting in a slight contraction. Hold for 1–2 seconds.

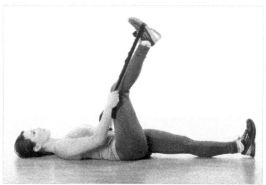

STRETCH: Breathe out as you slowly pull the strap with both hands so that your right foot moves toward your head while maintaining the slight bent-leg position. Stretch for 2 seconds.

Repeat as needed, then switch sides.

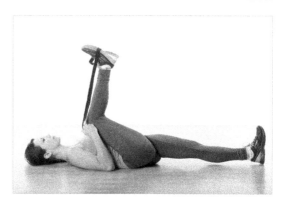

Lying Popliteus

Target: Hamstring muscles

START: Lie on your back with both legs straight. Secure your right foot into a loop of the strap and grasp the ends of the strap with both hands around knee level. Extend your right leg to the ceiling.

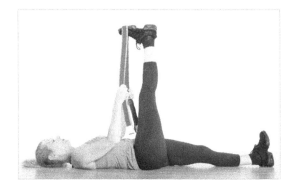

CONTRACT: While maintaining a straight leg, slowly pull on the strap to bring your right leg toward your head. Once the leg has reached a stretched position, slowly push the ball of your foot up against the strap. Hold for 1–2 seconds.

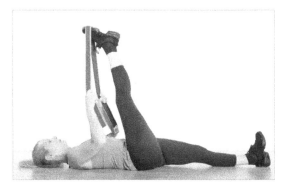

STRETCH: Breathe out as you slowly pull the strap down toward the ground, causing the toes to point toward the ground via ankle dorsiflexion. This will result in a stretch that will be felt behind the knee. Stretch for 2 seconds.

Repeat as needed, then switch sides.

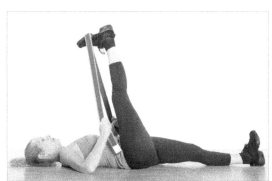

Standing Squat

Target: Lower back

START: Anchor the middle loop of the strap against an immobile object (nail, clip, post, etc.) at or slightly above head height. Standing upright with your body facing the anchor, grasp one end of the strap in each hand. From this position, take 1–3 steps back from the anchor position to increase the tension slightly on the strap. Stand with your feet shoulder-width apart with your toes pointing forward.

CONTRACT: Slowly bring both arms toward head height, increasing the contraction. Hold for 1–2 seconds.

STRETCH: Breathe out as you slowly shift your body weight down and squat down low while keeping your back straight, increasing the stretch throughout your back. Focus on pushing your weight through your heels and pressing the weight of your upper body through your glutes in a down and backward direction. Hold for 2 seconds.

Repeat as needed.

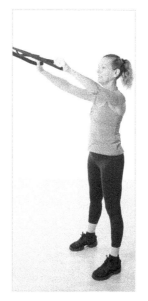

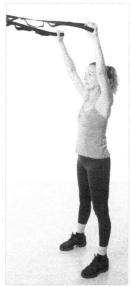

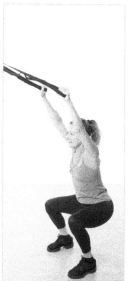

Standing Sumo Squat

Target: Lower back, hips

START: Anchor the middle loop of the strap against an immobile object (nail, clip, post, etc.) above head height. Standing upright with your body facing the anchor, grasp one end of the strap in each hand. Take 1–3 steps back from the anchor to increase the tension slightly on the strap. Stand with your feet wider than shoulder width apart with toes pointed outward.

CONTRACT: Increase the tension in the glutes and legs with an isometric contraction. Hold for 1–2 seconds.

STRETCH: Breathe out as you slowly shift your body weight down and squat low to the ground while keeping your back straight, increasing the stretch throughout the lower back and hips. Focus on pushing your weight through your heels and pressing the weight of your upper body through your glutes in a down and backward direction. Hold for 2 seconds.

Repeat as needed.

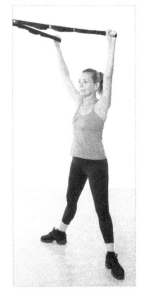

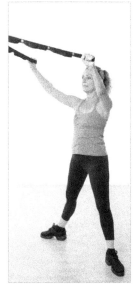

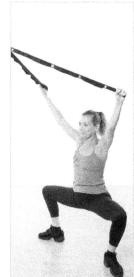

Standing Swan Dive

Target: Lower back, hamstrings

START: Anchor the middle loop of the strap against an immobile object (nail, clip, post, etc.) above head level. Standing upright with your body facing the anchor, grasp one end of the strap in each hand. Take 1–3 steps back from the anchor to increase the tension slightly on the strap. Stand with both feet together.

CONTRACT: Slowly take both arms toward the side, forming a cross. Hold for 2 seconds.

STRETCH: Breathe out as you slowly bend at the hip, keeping your back straight with the goal of forming close to a 90-degree angle at your hips. This will increase the stretch through your lower back and hamstring muscles. Hold for 2 seconds.

Repeat as needed.

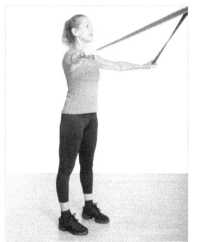

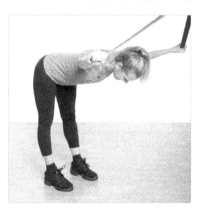

Standing Lunge & Rotation

Target: Quadriceps, glutes and lateral muscles of the trunk

START: Anchor the middle loop of the strap against an immobile object (nail, clip, post, etc.) at or slightly above head height. Standing upright with your body facing the anchor, grasp one end of the strap in each hand. Take 1–3 steps back from the anchor to increase the tension slightly on the strap. Step forward with your left foot into a forward lunge position with both knees bent at 90-degree angles. Keep your back straight.

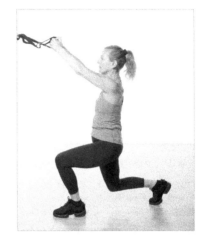

CONTRACT: With your hands above your head, slowly bring the strap backward toward your head, increasing the contraction. Hold for 2 seconds.

STRETCH: Breathe out as you slowly rotate your trunk toward the left while keeping your hips pointing forward, increasing rotational range of motion throughout the trunk. Hold for 2 seconds.

Repeat as needed, then switch sides.

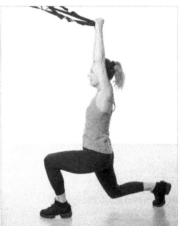

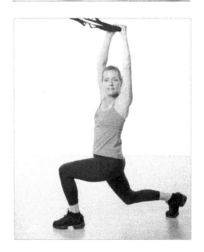

Standing Wiper Stretch (Lateral Flexion)

Target: Obliques, erector spinae, lower back

START: Anchor the middle loop of the strap against an immobile object (nail, clip, post, etc.) at or slightly above head height. Stand upright with your body perpendicular to the anchor, with the left side of your body closest to the anchor. Grasp the end of the strap with your right hand. Take 1–3 steps to your right, away from the anchor.

CONTRACT: Slowly bring your right arm above your head, increasing the contraction. Hold for 2 seconds.

STRETCH: Breathe out as you slowly shift your weight to your right side, pressing your right hip out to the right, increasing the stretch in the lateral flexor muscles of the right side of your lower back. To increase the stretch, take 1–2 more small steps to your right. Stretch for 2 seconds.

Repeat as needed, then switch sides.

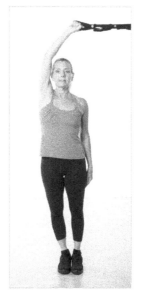

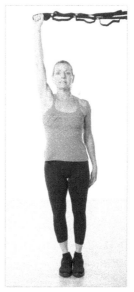

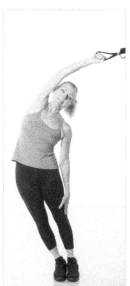

Kneeling Quad Stretch

Target: Quadriceps

START: Anchor the middle loop of the strap against an immobile object (nail, clip, post, etc.) above head height. Stand facing away from the anchor and grasp both ends of the strap with your left hand. Slowly drop your left knee to the ground (rest it on a towel or other soft surface if necessary) and keep your right leg in a lunge position, with your right foot firmly on the ground and your right knee bent 90 degrees.

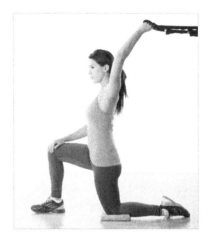

CONTRACT: Slowly bring your left arm above your head to slightly increase the contraction. Hold 1–2 seconds.

STRETCH: Breathe out as you simultaneously and slowly shift your left hip forward and move your left arm backward toward the anchor, increasing the stretch in your left hip flexor. To increase the stretch even further, take 1–2 steps away from the anchor. Stretch for 2 seconds.

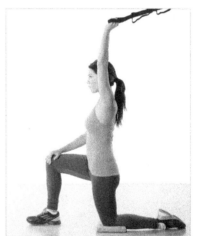

Repeat as needed, then switch sides.

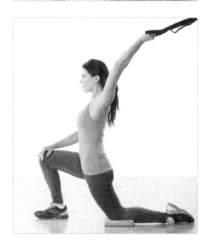

INDEX

ACKNOWLEDGMENTS

"From what we get, we can make a living;
what we give, however, makes a life."
—*Arthur Ashe*

Thousands of individuals have played an important role. The saying "it takes a village to raise a child" is very true. True thanks to my village of mentors, advisors, teachers, students, friends, critics, colleagues and family who have helped in unmeasurable ways. I want to acknowledge my parents (Paul and Sylvia) for the courage to go against the grain and the lifetime of lessons and love. Thanks also to my wife (Mary Jo) for keeping the balance and the constant love and support.

Stay flexible, my friends.

ABOUT THE AUTHOR

Mark Kovacs, Ph.D., FACSM, CSCS*D, CTPS, MTPS, is a sport scientist and human performance expert. He's the executive director of the International Tennis Performance Association (iTPA), the worldwide leader in tennis-specific performance, education and certification (www.itpa-tennis.org). He was a collegiate all-American and NCAA champion at Auburn University. After playing professional tennis, he pursued his graduate degree in exercise science with a Ph.D. in exercise physiology. Mark is a fellow of the American College of Sports Medicine, a certified strength and conditioning specialist through the National Strength and Conditioning Association, a certified health/fitness instructor through the American College of Sports Medicine, and a United States Track and Field Level II sprints coach, as well as a certified tennis coach. He's also a Master Tennis Performance Specialist (MTPS) through the iTPA. Mark has been published in numerous top scientific journals, presented at national and international conferences, and has been a keynote speaker on five continents. He has trained dozens of Olympic and professional athletes and was the assistant editor-in-chief of the *Strength and Conditioning Journal*. Previously he oversaw the sport science, coaching education, and strength-and-conditioning departments for the United States Tennis Association (USTA) and was also the Director of the Gatorade Sport Science Institute (GSSI). He has written five books on topics including dynamic stretching, recovery and tennis anatomy. He can be contacted through his personal website: www.mark-kovacs.com.

Printed in the USA
CPSIA information can be obtained
at www.ICGtesting.com
JSHW051422101223
53330JS00006B/51